SAMUEL HAHNEMANN'S

ORGANON

OF

HOMŒOPATHIC MEDICINE

Aude Sapere.

THIRD AMERICAN EDITION,

WITH IMPROVEMENTS AND ADDITIONS FROM THE LAST GERMAN EDITION,

AND

DR. C. HERING'S INTRODUCTORY REMARKS.

NEW-YORK:

WILLIAM RADDE, No. 322 BROADWAY
PHILADELPHIA: C. L. RADEMACHER, 239 ARCH-STREET.
BOSTON: OTIS CLAPP, 12 SCHOOL-STREET.
ST. LOUIS: FRANKSEN & WESSELHOEFT.

1849

H. Ludwig & Co., Printers,
70 Vesey-street.

SOME REMARKS

FOR THE THIRD AMERICAN EDITION OF HAHNEMANN'S ORGANON.

It is now twelve years since the first edition of the ORGANON OF MEDICINE appeared in this country. Since that period, the number of Homœopathic physicians in the United States has more than doubled every four years. This increase has been gradual, sometimes more, and at others less rapid, but always without interruption ; and at no time, neither in this country nor in Europe, has there been any retrogression from the ground gained. However, there have never been wanting those who asserted that Homœopathy was on the decline, and indeed was dead ; which reminds us of the old adage, that when a man is said to be dead, he has usually the promise of a long life. Other opponents have entertained great hopes, when they have learned that the adherents of our school are divided into different parties. This is like the friends of royalty in Europe, predicting the downfall of republican institutions in this country, because there are here various political parties. Among so large a number of physicians, it is quite natural that different opinions should be entertained and promulgated, and even that partisan conflicts should arise. But against the stubborn adherents of the old-school doctrines, these various parties stand united as the varied wings of one common army.

All Homœopathic physicians are united under the banner of the great law of cure, *similia similibus curantur ;* however they may differ in regard to the theoretical explanation of that law, or the extent to which it may be applied.

All Homœopathic physicians also acknowledge that provings upon the healthy are indispensable in ascertaining the unknown curative powers of drugs.

And finally : all Homœopaths concur in giving but one medicine at a time, never mixing different drugs together under the absurd expectation that each will act according to their dictum. This is the glorious tri-colour of our school, which will make the circuit of the world, and in these we are as the heart of one man.

It is not a little gratifying to find, that all the recent discoveries in Chemistry and Physiology, serve to confirm and establish the principles of our system, while they contradict the usual pathological opinions of the day. The wonderful discoveries in Pathological Anatomy, in ascertaining the material and chemical changes produced by disease and medicines, while they are a valuable addition to our knowledge, serve only to engender in the old school such doctrines as "Young Physic," according to which the patient is scientifically informed of the nature of his disorder, and gravely left to the efforts of nature. Even the Water Cure, is only the servant of the doctrine of Hahnemann, cleansing and renovating the house to be occupied by us.

While the various dissensions among the old school are favouring the extension of Homœopathy, the varied diversities among ourselves serve only to develop and advance our principles. What important influence can it exert, whether a Homœopath adopt the theoretical opinions of Hahnemann or not, so long as he holds fast the practical rules of the master, and the Materia Medica of our school? What influence can it have, whether a physician adopt or reject the Psora-theory, so long as he always selects the most similar medicine possible? Even in the larger or smaller doses, the masses or the potences, allowing that there is a great difference between them according to the testimony of the friends of each, yet all this difference dwindles into insignificance, when we compare the results of Homœopathic with that of common Allopathic practice. Hence we may console ourselves, leaving to farther researches to confirm or rectify Hahnemann's theory of potences, and to establish a rule without exceptions, according to which, the lower or the higher potences shall be the most appropriate in each individual case. There will always be a large number of physicians who either do not understand, or will not learn, how to select for each particular case the one only proper medicine, and such will always find it most comfortable to employ massive doses. There will always be perhaps as large a number, on the other hand, who will by and by know how to hit the nail upon the head, and they will learn to prefer the high potences. Even Hahnemann himself required more than a score of years to learn this. As through war we come to the possession of peace, so in the world of science, through conflict and trial, we come to the possession of truth. It was an old motto of Luther's,

"Lass die Geister auf einander platzen."

CONSTANTINE HERING.

Philadelphia, November 1, 1848.

ADVERTISEMENT.

One of the first occasions which led to the publication of the present edition of the Organon, was the express desire of Hahnemann that an enlarged and improved English version of it, from the fifth German edition, might appear in the United States. With the view of fulfilling, as much as possible, every just demand, the Academy entrusted the revision of the following work to several gentlemen, and would here express their particular obligations to Constantine Hering, M. D., Charles F. Matlack, M. D., of Philadelphia, and to Messrs. J. Radcliffe and A. Bauer, for services rendered in its preparation.

JNO. ROMIG, M. D.,
Chairman of the Board of Directors.

Academy of the Homœopathic Healing Art,
Allentown, Pa., October, 1836.

PREFACE TO THE BRITISH EDITION.

An accidental interview with a Russian physician, in the year 1828, made me acquainted for the first time with the medical doctrine of homœopathy; the principle of which is, that certain medicines, when administered internally in a healthy state of the system, produce certain effects, and that the same medicines are to be used when symptoms similar to those which they give rise to occur in disease. This doctrine, directly opposite to that which hitherto formed the basis of medical practice in these countries, attracted my attention. I immediately procured Hahnemann's Materia Medica Pura, in which the doctrine is partially explained, with the view of investigating the system experimentally, and reporting my observations thereon, free from theory, prejudice, or party. The first inquiry was, whether the proposition *similia similibus curantur* was true. This investigation was confined to a single substance at a time. To ascertain the effects of sulphate of quinine, healthy individuals were selected, to whom grain doses of the medicine were administered three times a day. After using it for some days, stomach-sickness, loss of appetite, a sense of cold along the course of the spine, rigour, heat of skin, and general perspiration, succeeded. Effects similar to these are often observed when this medicine is injudiciously selected in the treatment of disease. It sometimes happens, that the symptoms of ague are aggravated by the prolonged use of sulphate of quinia, and soon after it is withdrawn, the disease gradually subsides. The result of experiments and observations on this remedy elucidate its homœopathic action.

Mercurial preparations, when administered internally, produce symptoms local and constitutional, so closely resembling the poison of lues venerea, that medical practitioners, who have spent many years in the investigation of syphilis, find it very difficult—nay, in some instances impossible, (guided by the appearances,)—to distinguish one disease from the other. Of all the medicines used in the treatment of lues, mercury is the only one that has stood the test of time and experience. Let us then compare the effects of syphilis with those of mercury :—The venereal poison produces on the skin pustules, scales, and tubercles. Mercury produces directly the same defœdations of the skin. Syphilis excites inflammation of the periosteum, and caries of the bones. Mercury does the same. Inflammation of the iris from lues is an every-day occurrence ; the same disease is a very frequent consequence of mercury. Ulceration of the throat is a common symptom in syphilis ; the same affection results from mercury. Ulcers on the organs of reproduction are the result of both the poison and the remedy, and furnish another proof of the doctrine *similia similibus*.

Nitric acid is generally recommended in cutaneous diseases ; the internal use of this remedy, in a very dilute form, produces scaly eruptions over the surface of the body ; and the external application of a solution, in the proportion of one part acid to one hundred and twenty-eight parts of water, will produce inflammation and ulceration of the skin. These observations would lead to the conclusion, that nitric acid cures cutaneous diseases by the faculty it possesses of producing a similar disease of the skin. Nitrate of potash, administered internally in small doses, produces a frequent desire to pass water, accompanied with pain and heat. When this state of the urinary system exists as a consequence of disease, or the application of a blister, a very dilute solution of the same remedy has been found beneficial.

The ordinary effects of hyoscyamus niger are, vertigo, delirium, stupefaction, and somnolency. Where one or other of these diseased states exists, it yields to small doses of the tincture of this plant. The internal use of hyoscyamus is followed by mental aberration, the leading features of which are jealousy and irascibility. When these hallucinations exist, this remedy is indicated.

Opium in general causes drowsiness, torpor, and deep sleep, and yet this remedy in small doses removes these symptoms when they occur in disease

Sulphur is a specific against itch; notwithstanding which, when it is administered to healthy individuals, it frequently excites a pustular eruption, resembling itch in every particular.

These observations corroborate the statements of our author as to the value and importance of homœopathy; and were not the limits of a preface too confined, I could bring forward the actual experiments from which these deductions have been drawn.

On the subject of small doses of medicines, a few observations will suffice.

A mixture composed of one drop of hydrocyanic acid and eight ounces of water, administered in a drachm dose, has produced vertigo and anxious breathing. Vomiting has followed the use of the sixteenth of a grain of emetic tartar; narcotism, the twentieth of a grain of muriate of morphia; and spirit of ammonia, in doses of one drop, acts on the system as a stimulant.

On the homœopathic attenuation of medicines, many are sceptical, and presume that the quantity of the article extant in the dose, cannot produce a medicinal effect. I refer to the pages of the Organon for an elucidation of this proposition, and will relate an experiment, which may serve to explain the degree of dilution substances are capable of. One grain of nitrate of silver, dissolved in 1560 grains of distilled water, to which were added two grains of muriatic acid, a gray precipitate of chloride of silver was evident in every part of the liquor. One grain of iodine dissolved in a drachm of alcohol, and mixed with the same quantity of water as in the preceding experiment, to which were added two grains of starch, dissolved in an ounce of water, caused an evident blue tint in the solution. In these experiments, the grain of the nitrate of silver and iodine must have been divided into $\frac{1}{15120}$ of a grain.

A few particulars connected with the discoverer and founder of the homœopathic system of medicine cannot but prove interesting to the readers of this volume. SAMUEL HAHNEMANN was born in 1755, at Misnia, in Upper Saxony. He exhibited at an early age traits of a superior genius; his school education being completed, he applied himself to the study of natural philosophy and natural history, and afterwards prosecuted the study of medicine at Leipsic, and other universities. A most accurate observer, a skilful experimenter, and an indefatigable searcher after truth, he appeared formed by nature for the investigation and improvement of medical science. On commencing the study of medicine, he soon became disgusted with the mass of contradictory assertions and theories which then existed. He found everything in this department obscure, hypothetical, and vague, and resolved to abandon the medical profession. Having been previously engaged in the study of chemistry, he determined on translating into his native language the best English and French works on the subject. Whilst engaged in translating the Materia Medica of the illustrious Cullen, in 1790, in which the febrifuge virtues of cinchona bark are described, he became fired with the desire of ascertaining its mode of action. Whilst in the enjoyment of the most robust health, he commenced the use of this substance, and in a short time was attacked with all the symptoms of intermittent fever, similar in every respect to those which that medicine is known to cure. Being struck with the identity of the two diseases, he immediately divined the great truth which has become the foundation of the new medical doctrine of homœopathy.

Not contented with one experiment, he tried the virtues of

medicines on his own person, and on that of others. In his investigations he arrived at this conclusion: that the substance employed possessed an inherent power of exciting in healthy subjects the same symptoms which it is said to cure in the sick. He compared the assertions of ancient and modern physicians upon the properties of poisonous substances with the result of his own experiments, and found them to coincide in every respect; and upon these deductions he brought forth his doctrine of homœopathy. Taking this law for a guide, he recommenced the practice of medicine, with every prospect of his labours being ultimately crowned with success.

In 1796 he published his first dissertation on homœopathy in Hufeland's Journal. A treatise on the virtues of medicine appeared in 1805, and the "*Organon*" in 1810. Hahnemann commenced as a public medical teacher in Leipsic. in 1811, where, with his pupils, he zealously investigated the effects of medicines on the living body, which formed the basis of the Materia Medica Pura which appeared during the same year. Like many other discoverers in medicine, the author of the Organon has been persecuted with the utmost rigour; and in 1820 he quitted his native country in disgust. In retirement he was joined by several of his pupils, who formed themselves into a society for the purpose of prosecuting the homœopathic system of physic, and reporting their observations thereon. Several fasciculi detailing their labours have been since published.

In 1824 the homœopathic doctrine was embraced by Rau, physician to the Duke of Hesse Darmstadt; by Bigelius, physician to the Emperor of Russia; by Stegemann, and many other names celebrated in medicine.

We find, from a published letter o Dr. Peschier of Geneva, that Hahnemann resides at Cœthen, (capital of Anhalt-Cœthen,) in the enjoyment of perfect health and spirits. He is consulted by patients from almost every nation, who have been attracted by his fame as a physician.

Of the doctrine of homœopathy generally, I have little more to add in this place; time will develop the truth or fallacy of the principle on which it is founded; but in the mean time let us not lose sight of the fact, that this new system of physic is spreading throughout the continent of Europe with the rapidity of lightning. Germany, Austria, Russia, and Poland, have already done homage to the doctrine, and physicians have been appointed to make a specific trial of its effects, the results of which are unequivocally acknowledged to be of a favourable nature. The writings of the illustrious Hahnemann have appeared in five different languages, independent of the present version of his "Organon;" and in France alone, a translation of this work, from the pen of A. J. L. Jourdan, member of the Academie Royale de Medecine, has reached a fourth edition.

Convinced, from reflection and observation, of the value of homœopathy, the first step in the propagation and dissemination of this doctrine, in Britain, was to obtain an English version of the " Organon."

SAMUEL STRATTEN.

Dublin, June 14th, 1833.

PREFACE TO THE FIRST AMERICAN EDITION.

FIRST impressions commonly determine our judgment of books as well as men. If, on a first interview, a person be repulsive to us, and those who for years have had familiar intercourse with him, admit that we are excusable for first impressions, but nevertheless assure us that he is possessed of very valuable qualities, and that a nearer acquaintance with him may be useful to us,—when, in addition, our informants give us a key to a more correct judgment,—we are no longer justifiable in maintaining our original impressions. Still more would our opinions be influenced, if, before seeing the person, we were furnished in advance with a short and impartial representation of his character by one who knew him intimately. If this rule of judgment be applicable to persons, wherefore should it not apply to books?

The Organon contains much that is peculiar and different from the views hitherto entertained by the prevailing school of medicine. Most readers of the medical profession, therefore, conceive prejudices against it, and fall into the vulgar error of rejecting the whole, merely because they do not justly regard it as a whole,—they reject the main propositions, because they are offended at the subordinate.

The reader needs no elaborate introduction to the following work, and it is requisite, perhaps, only to apprise him of the different classes into which its several paragraphs may be divided; and this being done, we shall submit each separate class to his own judgment.

The entire contents of the Organon may be easily arranged under the four following divisions, which, indeed, do not occur in the order in which they are here given, but they might

easily have been designated in accordance to it, by causing
them to be severally printed in a different type. They consist,—1. Of discoveries—experimental propositions, or the results of actual experiment. 2. Of directions or instructions.
3. Of theoretical and philosophical illustrations. 4. Of de-
fences and accusations.

I.—OF DISCOVERIES.

Among men of deliberate and acute reflection, no difference
of opinion can exist relative to the truth of a discovery which
rests upon the basis of actual experiment. When the author
appeals to such experiments, they must be led to a repetition
of them, and not oppose their own opinions to the dictates of
experience; in fine, they have no other way in forming a
judgment, than that of accurate and careful experiment.

It may be said that every charlatan, in extolling his nostrums,
in like manner appeals to experience, and no one is required
for that reason to investigate the merits of his compounds;
but it will not be denied that, although the person of the
quack may deserve little forbearance; yet the remedy with
which he dupes the public may, in some cases, prove beneficial. The old school has received many remedies, mercury
among others, from the hands of the quack.

But, in the Organon, experience is not referred to for the
purpose of lauding any individual remedy; far more, it has
relation to an entire method of cure. None but a vulgar
dealer in calumny of the grosser sort, would attempt to de-
grade Hahnemann to a level with the charlatan; because he
promulgates his views and the peculiarities of his method, as
a learned physician, and in a manner that is sanctioned by
custom, and fully recognised in the history of medicine.

But his method, as we have already intimated, appeals to
experience. Not to mention the example of Brown, we need
only refer to that of Broussais, and the reports received strikingly in favour of his doctrines, or even to the contra-stimulus

of the Italians, which incessantly appeals to the same experience as the test of its value.

It is, indeed, desirable that every learned physician—professors, hospital physicians, and others in prominent stations—should carefully study, and, so far as the experiments are innocuous, prove his new method; nay, Hahnemann and his adherents often and ardently desire that every physician would learn, investigate, and prove homœopathy for himself.

But homœopathy is not only a new method, but much more.

This method does not rest upon new views, like every other hitherto promulgated, but *upon new discoveries, which appertain to the departments of natural philosophy*, the natural sciences, physiology and biology.

The doctrine that every peculiar substance—every mineral, plant, animal, in fact every part of them, or every preparation derived from a preceding one, produces a series of peculiar effects upon the human organism, manifestly belongs to the natural sciences, and only so far to the materia medica as the latter calls these properties into requisition. But it is a science in itself—a science which treats of the effect of a diversity of substances upon the human frame. Whether such a science, in point of fact, be capable of formation, and whether it have any value, can be determined only by experiment. It were equally foolish to deny this without trial, as it was formerly to deny, without exploring, the way which Columbus opened to the west. It would be inexcusable, in the present condition of the materia medica, confessedly imperfect, and deficient in all the attributes of a science, to despise this new way of Hahnemann, before knowing, by careful experiment, that it conducts to nothing better.

The doctrine of the preparation of the remedies into the so-called dilutions, belongs to natural philosophy, in common with the doctrines of magnetism, electricity, and galvanism. Nor is it more a subject of wonder than the latter—except that these sooner came under investigation by the natural philosopher.   The repetition of the new electro-magnetic experiments requires great accuracy; those concerning the operation of minute doses require just as much, nay, even more. To deny the results of the electro-magnetic experiments, previous to repeating them, were ridiculous, and it is equally so to deny the results of these.   But no hasty, superficial, partial, or wholly perverted experiments, must be instituted.

The doctrine that such dilutions or potences are capable of curing diseases according to the law " similia similibus," is a proposition which belongs to biology, and there finds its confirmation ; it likewise can only be investigated by experiment, and cannot be estimated without it.

The cautious investigator will not pass judgment upon all these discoveries, until he shall have performed a series of rigorous experiments.   Then only will he be prepared either to reject or accept the method founded thereon, or, at least, learn the useful part of it.

H.—DIRECTIONS.

These appertain to the method of cure, are derived from the long-continued application of the law previously referred to, and acquire their principal value from its truth.   No one can judge of them but he who has tested the truth of the experimental propositions, and in doing so, adhered to these directions.   By this means only can he become convinced of their great value, which is entirely lost on those who deny the discoveries.

We enumerate under this head, directions for the examination of the sick, for the preparation of the medicines, for trying them on the healthy subject, for the selection of the remedies, dietetics, and directions for the psychical treatment.

III.—ILLUSTRATIONS.

Hahnemann has appended certain theories to the laws of nature discovered by him, by which these laws are illustrated

and brought into unison with other laws already acknowledged, or with other theories received as true. This has never
been reckoned a subject of reproach to any discoverer. Man
will and must seek to illustrate the phenomena which he observes, and bring individual parts into co-aptation—the new
into harmony with that previously known. In this endeavour,
not only is he liable to err, but actually does err in the great
majority of cases; accordingly, few hypotheses and attempts
at explanation have endured long, and it is a fact of daily ac-
knowledgment, that one hypothesis gives place to another in
all sciences. Columbus himself entertained numerous conjectures which time has verified or overthrown. Whether the
theories of Hahnemann are destined to endure a longer or
a shorter space, whether they be the best or not, time only
can determine ; be it as it may, however, *it is a matter
of minor import* ce. For myself, I am generally considered
as a disciple a   adherent of Hahnemann, and I do indeed
declare, that I   n one among the most enthusiastic in doing homage to h   greatness ; but nevertheless I declare also,
that since my first acquaintance with homœopathy, (in the year
1821,) down to the present day, I have never yet accepted a
single theory in the Organon as it is there promulgated.   I feel
no aversion to acknowledge this even to the venerable sage
himself.   It is the genuine Hahnemannean spirit totally to disregard all theories, even those of one's own fabrication, when
they are in opposition to the results of pure experience.   All
theories and hypotheses have no positive weight whatever,
only so far as they lead to new experiments, and afford a better survey of the results of those already made.

Whoever, therefore, will assail the theories of Hahnemann,
or even altogether reject them, is at perfect liberty to do so;
but let him not imagine that he has thereby accomplished a
memorable achievement.   In every respect it is an affair of
little importance.

2

IV.—DEFENCES.

Opinions upon this head are also things of secondary consideration, inasmuch as the entire polemical matter is of subordinate estimation in forming a judgment concerning new discoveries. Had Hahnemann the right to defend himself as he has done, and thereby promote the progress of his doctrine, or had he not? We cannot judge concerning it, but justly commit the decision of the question to future history. The entire polemical part may be stricken out, without in the slightest degree changing the principal matters, or without having any influence either to ratify or invalidate the doctrine itself.

Is there a physician who feels that individual expressions will apply to him, let him take heed to the truth; but if they do not reach him, then is he unaffected by them. He who is offended at the polemical part, let him reflect that it is the first step towards an unjust estimate of the rest.

A just judgment is all that we wish from every reader of the Organon, and to contribute something to this end was the design of these preliminary remarks.

CONSTANTINE HERING.

Academy, Allentown, Penn., August 10, 1836.

CONTENTS.

INTRODUCTION.

ORGANON OF MEDICINE.

INTRODUCTION.

FROM the earliest period of time, mankind have been liable to disease, individually and collectively, arising from causes natural and moral. In the rude and simple forms of primitive life, few maladies appeared, and little skill was requisite to remove them; but as society became more dense, and men formed themselves into states, diseases multiplied, and medical aid became, in the same degree, necessary.

Thenceforward, at least after the days of Hippocrates, during a lapse of nearly two thousand five hundred years, men have fondly supposed, that these multiplied and complicated maladies were to be removed by methods originating purely in scheming and conjecture. Innumerable opinions on the nature and cure of diseases, have successively been promulgated; each distinguishing his own theory with the title of *system*, though directly at variance with every other, and inconsistent with itself.

Each of these refined productions dazzled the reader at first with its unintelligible display of wisdom, and attracted to the system-builder crowds of adherents, echoing his unnatural sophistry, but from which none of them could derive any improvement in the art of healing, until a new system, frequently in direct opposition to the former, appeared, supplanting it, and for a season acquiring celebrity. Yet none were in harmony with nature and experience—mere theories spun out of a refined imagination, from apparent consequences, which, on account of their subtilty and contradictions, were practically inapplicable at the bedside of the patient, and only fitted for idle disputation.

By the side of these theories, but unconnected with them all, a mode of cure was contrived, with medical substances of unknown quality compounded together, applied to diseases arbitrarily classified, and arranged in reference to their materiality, called *Allœopathia.* The pernicious results of such a practice, at variance with nature and experience, may be easily imagined.

Without seeking to detract from the reputation which many physicians have justly acquired by their skill in the sciences auxiliary to medicine, such as Natural Philosophy, Chemistry, Natural History in all its branches, and that of man in particular, Anthropology, Physiology, Anatomy, &c., &c., I shall occupy myself here with the practical part of Medicine only, in order to show the imperfect manner in which diseases have been treated till the present day. It is also far from my intention to pursue that mechanical routine by which the precious lives of our fellow-creatures are treated according to pocket-book recipes, volumes of which are still daily appearing before the public, and show, alas! how frequently, and to what extent, they are resorted to even at the present time. I turn from these, as undeserving of notice, and as a lasting reproach to the Faculty of Medicine. I shall merely speak of the Medical Art, such as it has existed till the present day, and which, on account of its antiquity, is supposed to be founded upon scientific principles.

It was the boast of the former schools of medicine, that their doctrine alone deserved the title of *"rational art of healing,"* because it was pretended that they alone sought after and removed the *morbid cause,* and *followed the traces of Nature herself in diseases.*

Tolle causam! cried they continually; but that was all : they seldom went farther than that vain exclamation. *They talked* of being able to discover the cause of disease, without succeeding in their pretended attempts; for, by far the greater number of diseases being of dynamic origin, as well as of a dynamic nature, and their cause, therefore, not admitting of discovery to the senses, they were reduced to the necessity of inventing one. By comparing, on the one hand, the normal state of the parts of the dead human body (anatomy) with the visible changes which those parts had undergone in subjects that had died of disease, (pathological anatomy,) and on the other, the functions of the living body, (physiology,) with the endless aberrations to which they are subject in the various stages of disease, (semeiotics, pathology,) and drawing from thence conclusions, relative to the invisible manner in which the changes are brought about in the *interior* of man, when in a diseased state, they succeeded in forming an obscure and imaginary picture, which theoretic medicine regarded as the *prima causa morbi*,* which afterwards became the *nearest cause*, and, at the same time, the *immediate essence of the disease*, and even the *disease itself;* although common sense tells us, that the cause of anything can never be, at the same time, both the cause and the thing itself.

How was it then possible, without deceiving themselves, to pretend to cure this yet undiscovered internal cause, or venture to prescribe for it medicines, whose curative tendency was equally for the most part unknown to them, and more especially, to mix up several of those unknown substances in what we term prescriptions?

However, the sublime project of discovering, *a priori*, some internal invisible cause of disease, resolved itself (at least among some self-conceited physicians of the old school) into a search,

---

* It would have been far more suitable to the good sense of mankind, and to the nature of the case, had they, in order to cure, attempted to discover, as the *causa morbi*, the originating cause of the disease itself, and had applied a method of treatment which they had found available for diseases springing from that originating cause, and for others of a like origin. For example, the same hydrargyrum is properly applied to every ulcer on the glans penis, after an impure coition, as hitherto with every venereal chancre—if they, I say, had discovered the originating cause of every other chronic (non-venereal) disease, either from a recent or a former infection in a psoric miasm; if for all these they had found a method of cure, with a therapeutic reference to each particular case, by which the whole and each separate chronic case could have been healed; then might they with justice have gained renown, that they in the treatment of chronic diseases were familiar with the *only useful* and successful *causa morborum chronicorum*, (*non venereorum*,) and adopting it as a basis, were capable of treating such cases with the best results. But they were incapable of curing the numberless chronic diseases in ages past, as their psoric origin was unknown to them, (a discovery which the world owes to homœopathia, as well as for an effectual method of treatment which it has provided,) and notwithstanding their vaunting that they alone had the *primam causam* in view in their proceeding; after all their boasted science, they had not the remotest suspicion of their psoric origin, and consequently every chronic disease has been mangled.

guided onward by the symptoms, after that which they might
presume to be the generic character of the existing malady.*
They endeavoured to find out whether it was spasm, debility,
or paralysis, fever or inflammation, induration or obstruction,
in some one of the parts ; excess of blood, (plethora,) or increase or deficiency of oxygen, carbon, hydrogen, or nitrogen,
in the fluids ; exaltation or depression of vitality in the arterial, venous, or capillary system ; a defect of relative proportion in the *factors* of sensibility, of irritability, or of nutrition.
These conjectures, honoured by the existing school with the
name of *Causal Indication*, and regarded by them as the only
rational part of medicine, were too hypothetical and fallacious
to be of any permanent utility in practice, and insufficient
(even if they had any just foundation) to point out the best
remedy in any particular case of disease. It is true, they
were flattering to the self-love of the learned inventor, but
acting on them only led him farther astray, and showed that
there was more of ostentation in the pursuit than any reason- ·
able hope of being able to profit by it, or arrive at the real curative indication.

How often has it occurred, that spasm or paralysis appeared to be in one part of the system, while inflammation seemed
to be in another !

On the other hand, where should we be able to procure certain remedies against each of these pretended general charac-
ters of diseases ? There could be none, save those which are
termed *specifics*—that is to say, medicines homogeneous to the
morbid irritation, (now called homœopathic,) and whose application has been prohibited by the old school of medicine, as
being highly dangerous,† because experience proved that the

---

* Every physician adopting a treatment of such a general character, however unblushingly he may affect to be an homœopathist, is and will always
remain a generalizing allœopathist, as without the most special individualiza-
tion, homœopathia has no meaning.

† " In cases where experience had revealed the homœopathic efficacy of
medicines, whose mode of operation, however, was inexplicable, the physicians made use of them, and relieved themselves from all further embarrassment by declaring them to be *specific*. Thus, by an unmeaning name that
was applied to them, all necessity for further reflection was superseded. But
homogeneous excitements—that is to say, specifics or homœopathics—had, for a
long time previously, been forbidden, as exercising an extremely dangerous influence." *Rau, Ueber das homœop. Heilverfahren, Heidelberg*, 1824, p.101, 102.

use of them in such powerful doses as had been usually administered was pernicious in maladies where the aptitude to undergo homœogeneous irritation existed to a great extent. Besides this, the old school never once thought of administering those medicines in very small or in extremely minute doses. Thus, no one ventured to cure in the direct and most natural way, by using homœogeneous and specific medicines, nor was it possible to do so, because the fullest extent of their effects was unknown, and in that state remained ; and had it been otherwise, it would have been impossible to have guessed out remedies so very applicable by such generalizing opinions.

However, the old school of medicine, aware that it was more consistent with reason to pursue a straightforward path than attempt a circuitous one, still imagined they could arrest disease by a *removal of the supposed morbid material cause.* In the theoretic researches after the image which they were to form to themselves of the disease, as well as in their pursuit of the curative indication, it was almost impossible for them to divest themselves of this idea of materiality, or be induced to consider the nature not only of material but spiritual organism, as being so potent in itself that the changes in its sensations and vital movements (which are called diseases) are principally, and almost solely, the result of dynamic influence, and could not be produced by any other cause.

The old school regarded all the solids and fluids which had become changed by disease, (those in-normal substances, turgescent or secreted,) as the exciting cause of the disorder; or, at least, on account of their supposed reaction, they were considered to be the cause which kept up disease, and this latter opinion is adhered to, even at the present day.

This theory first inspired them with the idea of accomplishing causal cure, by using every means in their power to expel from the body that imaginary and supposed material cause of disease. Hence arises the continual practice of evacuating bile in cases of bilious fever* by emetics,—the system of pre-

---

* The Court Physician, Rau, (*loc. cit.*, p. 176,) at a time when he was not yet fully initiated into homœopathic medicine, but when, however, he entertained a perfect conviction of the dynamic origin of these fevers, was in the habit of curing them without any evacuating medicines whatever, merely by one or two small doses of homœopathic medicines. In his work, he relates two remarkable instances of cure.

scribing vomits in the so-named foul stomach,*—the diligence
in purging away mucus and intestinal worms, where there is
paleness of the countenance, ravenous appetite, pains in the

* In a sudden affection of the stomach, with frequent nauseous eructations,
as of spoiled food, (sulphuretted hydrogen,) accompanied with depression of
mind, cold at the feet, hands, &c., physicians, till the present time, were in
the habit of attending only to the degenerated contents of the stomach. A
powerful emetic *must* fetch it out entirely. This object was usually effected
by the use of tartrate of antimony, with or without a mixture of ipecacuanha.
But did the patient recover his health as soon as he had vomited ? No! these
gastric affections of dynamic origin are commonly produced by a disturbed
state of mind, (grief, fright, anger,) cold, exertion of the mind or body immediately after eating, and sometimes even after a temperate enjoyment of food.
Neither the tartrate of antimony, nor the ipecacuanha, are suited to the purpose of removing this dynamic aberration, and the revolutionary vomiting
which they excite is equally unserviceable. Besides provoking a manifestation of the symptoms of disease, they strike one blow more at the health of
the patient, and the secretion of bile becomes deranged ; so that if the patient
did not happen to be of a robust constitution before, he must feel greatly indisposed for *several* days after the pretended causal cure, notwithstanding the
violent expulsion of the entire contents of the stomach. But if, instead of
those powerful and oft injurious evacuating medicines, the patient should
only smell once to a globule of sugar the size of a mustard seed, impregnated
with the thirtieth dilution of pulsatilla, which infallibly restores the order and
harmony of the whole system, and that of the stomach in particular, then he
is cured in the space of two hours. If any eructations still take place, they
are nothing more than air, without taste or smell ; the contents of the stomach are no longer vitiated, and at the next meal the patient recovers his accustomed appetite, his health, and his air of repose. This is what ought to
be denominated " real cure," because it has destroyed the cause. The other
is an imaginary one, and only fatigues and does injury to the patient.

Even a stomach overloaded with indigestible food *never* requires a medicinal emetic. In such a case, nature knows full well how to disencumber herself of the excess, by the spontaneous vomitings which she excites, and
which may at all times be aided by mechanical provocation, such as tickling
the fauces. By this means we avoid the accessary effects which result from
the operation of emetics, and a little coffee (without milk) afterwards suffices
to hasten the passage of any matters into the intestines, which the stomach
may still contain.

But if, after having been filled beyond measure, the stomach does not possess, or has lost the irritability necessary to produce spontaneous vomiting ;
and the patient, tormented by acute pain of the epigastrium, does not experience the slightest desire to vomit, in such a state an emetic would only
cause a dangerous or mortal inflammation of the intestines ; whereas, slight
and repeated doses of a strong infusion of coffee, would reanimate the de-

stomach, or intumescence of the belly in children,* the letting of blood in cases of hemorrhage,† and especially bleeding of all kinds,‡ as their chief indication in inflammatory cases, and,

pressed irritability of the stomach, and place it in a condition to evacuate of itself, either upwards or downwards, the substances contained in its interior, however considerable the quantity may have been. Here, again, the treatment which ordinary physicians pretend to direct against the cause, is out of place.

It is the custom, at the present day, when gastric acid becomes superabundant, (which is frequently the case in chronic diseases,) to administer an emetic to relieve the stomach of its presence. But the following morning, or a few days after, the stomach contains just the same quantity, if not more. On the other hand, the pains cease of themselves, when their dynamic cause is attacked by an extremely small dose of dilute sulphuric acid, or with another antipsoric remedy, homœopathic with the various symptoms. It is thus that, in the plans of treatment, which the old school say are directed against the morbific cause, the favourite object is to expel with trouble, and to the great detriment of the patient, the material product of the dynamic disorder, without exerting themselves in the least to find out the dynamic source of the evil, in order to vanquish it homœopathically, as well as to annihilate everything that might emanate from it, and thus treat the disease in a *rational manner.*

* Symptoms that depend solely upon a psoric diathesis, and which easily yield to (dynamic) mild antipsoric remedies, without either emetics or purgatives.

† Though most morbid hemorrhages depend solely on a dynamic change of the vital powers, still the old school assign a superabundance of blood as their cause, and never fail to prescribe bleeding, in order to relieve the body of this supposed excess of the juice of life. The disastrous consequences which frequently result from this mode of treatment, such as prostration of the powers, tendency to, and even typhoid state itself, they ascribe to the malignity of the disease, *which they are then often unable to subdue :* in short, though the patient may fall a sacrifice, they, nevertheless, consider that they have acted in conformity to the adage, *causam tolle;* that is, according to their common remark, " We have done everything that could possibly be done —let the consequence now be what it may !! "

‡ Though the living human body may, perhaps, never have contained one drop of blood too much, still the old school regard a supposed plethora, or superabundance of blood, as the principal material cause of hemorrhages and inflammations, and which ought to be attacked by bleeding, cupping, and leeches. This they call a treatment of the cause, and a rational mode of proceeding. In fevers with an inflammatory character, as well as in acute pleurisy, they even go so far as to regard the coagulable lymph that exists in the blood, (and which they call the buffy coat,) as the peccant matter, which they do their best to evacuate, as much as possible, by repeated bleedings,

in imitation of a blood-thirsty physician of Paris, the application to the parts affected of a frequently fatal number of
leeches.   By this mode of proceeding, they think they pursue

although it often occurs that this crust becomes thicker and tougher in appearance at every fresh emission of blood.   In this manner, when inflammatory fever cannot be subdued, they often bleed the patient till he is near death,
in order to remove this buffy coat, or the pretended plethora, without ever
suspecting that the inflamed blood is nothing more than the product of the
acute fever, the inflammatory immaterial (dynamic) irritation ; and that this
latter, the sole cause of the disturbance that has taken place in the vascular
system, may be arrested by a homœopathic remedy ; such, for example, as a
globule of sugar impregnated with the juice of aconite of the decillionth degree of dilution, avoiding the vegetable acids ; so that the *most violent pleu-
ritic fever*, with all its attendant alarming symptoms, is cured in the *space of
twenty-four hours at farthest, without loss of blood, or any antiphlogistic
whatever*, (if a little blood, by way of experiment, be now taken from the
vein, it will no longer exhibit any traces of inflammatory crust,) whereas, another patient, similar in every respect, and treated according to the pretended
rational mode of the old school, if he escape death after numerous bleedings
and unspeakable suffering, often languishes yet entire months, reduced and
exhausted, before he can stand upright, if he is not taken off in the interval
(as is frequently the case) by a typhus fever, a leucophlegmacy, or a pulmonary consumption, the common result of this mode of treatment.
   He who feels the steady pulse of a patient an hour before the shivering
comes on, which always precedes acute pleurisy, will be much surprised
when, two hours after, (the fever having set in,) they try to persuade him
that the violent plethora which then exists, makes repeated bleeding necessary ; and he asks himself, by what miracle could those pounds of blood, which
are now to be taken away, and which he had, two hours before, felt beating
with a tranquil movement, have effected an entrance into the arteries of the patient ?   There could not be an ounce of blood more in his veins than he possessed two hours before, when he was in good health.   Thus, when the allœopathic physician prescribes venesection, it is not at all superfluous blood that
he draws from the patient attacked with acute fever, because this liquid could
not possibly exist in too great quantity ; but he deprives him of a portion of
the normal blood necessary to his existence, and to the re-establishment of
health ;—a grievous loss, which it is no longer in his power to repair, and
he thinks, notwithstanding, to have acted according to the axiom *tolle causam*,
to which he gives so wrong an interpretation, whilst the sole and true cause
of the malady was, not a superabundance of blood, which could never exist,
but a dynamic inflammatory irritation of the vascular system, as is proved
by the permanent and speedy cure which may be effected in similar cases, by
administering one or two incredibly minute doses of the juice of aconite,
which is homœopathic with this irritation.   The old school err not less in
recommending partial bleedings, and still more so in the application of leeches

the causal indication, and treat the patient in a rational manner. They likewise suppose, that by removing a polypus by ligature, extirpating a tumefied gland, or destroying the same by suppuration, produced by local irritation, by dissecting out the insulated cyst of a steatomatous or meliceretous tumour, operating for aneurism, fistula lachrymalis, or fistula in ano, amputating a cancerous breast, or a limb where the bone had become carious, &c., &c., to have cured the maladies in a radical manner, and destroyed their cause. They imagine the same thing when they make use of their repellent remedies, and dry up old ulcers in the legs by astringents, oxides of lead, copper and zinc, accompanied, it is true, with purgatives, which only weaken, without diminishing the fundamental evil; when they cauterize chancres, destroy condylomata locally, drive back itch from the skin, by sulphur ointment, lead, mercury, or zinc; and, finally, when they cure opthalmia with solutions of lead or zinc, and drive away pain from the members by the use of opodeldoc, volatile liniment, or fumigations of cinnabar and amber. In all such cases, they think they have annihilated the evil, triumphed over the disease, and performed a rational treatment directed against the cause. *But mark what follows!* New forms of diseases, which infallibly manifest themselves sooner or later, and which, when they appear, are taken for fresh maladies, *being always worse than the primitive affection*, evidently refute the theories of the old school. These ought to undeceive them, and prove that the evil has an immaterial cause, the deeper concealed because its origin is dynamic, and it cannot be destroyed but by dynamic power.

———

in great numbers, when treating local inflammation after the manner of Broussais. The palliative relief which they afford at first, is not crowned by a rapid or perfect cure; the weakness and valetudinarian state to which the parts that have been thus treated, remain a prey, and sometimes even the whole body, sufficiently prove how erroneous it is to attribute local inflammation to local plethora; and how deceitful are the consequences of such bleedings when this inflammatory irritation, apparently local, can be destroyed in a prompt and permanent manner, by a small dose of aconite, or, according to circumstances, of belladonna, a mode by which the malady is speedily and effectively cured, without having recourse to bleedings, which nothing can justify.

An hypothesis, which the schools of medicine generally entertained until a recent date, (and, I might even say, until the present time,) is that of morbid or peccant matter in diseases, however subtile that matter may be supposed to be. The blood and lymphatic vessels were to be disencumbered of this matter by the exhalants, the skin, the kidneys, and the salivary glands; the chest was to be freed from it by the trachial and bronchial glands; the stomach and the intestinal canal by vomiting and alvine dejections—to be able to say that the body was cleansed of the material cause which excited the disease, and that they had accomplished a radical cure according to the principle—*tolle causam !*

By incisions made in the diseased body, in which, for years together, foreign substances are inserted, producing tedious ulcers, (issues and setons,) they would draw off the *materia peccans* from the (purely dynamically) diseased body, as dregs escape by a faucet from a filthy cask. By perpetual blisters, (cantharides and mezereum,) they also think to abstract this peccant matter, and thus thoroughly purify the system. By such inconsiderate and unnatural treatment, the exhausted patient is commonly brought into a condition totally incurable.

I grant it was more convenient for human incapacity to suppose, that in the maladies which presented themselves for cure, there existed some morbid principle, of which the mind could conceive the materiality, especially as the patients willingly lent themselves to an hypothesis of this kind. By admitting this, they had nothing further to do than to administer a sufficient quantity of medicines capable of purifying the blood and the fluids, of exciting urine and perspiration, promoting expectoration, and scouring out the stomach and intestines. This is the reason that all the authors on Materia Medica, who have appeared since Dioscorides up to the present day, say nothing of the peculiar and special action of individual medicines, but content themselves, after enumerating their supposed virtues in any particular case of disease, with saying, whether they promote urine, perspiration, expectoration, or the menstrual flow, and particularly if they have the effect of emptying the alimentary canal upwards or downwards, because the principal tendency of the efforts of practitioners has, at all times, been the expulsion of a morbid material principle, and of a quantity of acrid matter, which they imagine ! to be the cause of disease. ∕

These, however, were vague dreams, gratuitous suppositions, hypotheses destitute of foundation, skilfully invented for the convenience of therapeutic medicine, which flattered itself that it would have an easier task to perform in contending against morbid material principles. (*Si modo essent !*)

But the essence of diseases, and their cure, will not bend to our fancies and convenience ; diseases will not, out of deference to our stupidity, cease to be *dynamic aberrations, which our spiritual existence undergoes in its mode of feeling and acting,—that is to say, immaterial changes in the state of health.*

The causes of disease cannot possibly be material, since the least foreign substance* introduced into the blood-vessels, however mild it may appear to us, is suddenly repulsed by the vital power, as a poison ; or, where this does not take place, death itself ensues. Even when the smallest foreign particle chances to insinuate itself into any of the sensitive parts, the principle of life which is spread throughout our interior, does not rest until it has procured the expulsion of this body, by pain, fever, suppuration, or gangrene. And, in a skin disease of twenty years' standing, could this vital principle, whose activity is indefatigable, suffer patiently, during twenty years, an exanthemic material principle (the poison of tetter, scrofula or gout) to exist in the fluids ? What nosologist has ever seen one of those morbid principles, of which he speaks with so much confidence, and upon which he presumes to found a plan of medical treatment ? Who has ever been able to exhibit to the view, the principle of gout, or the virus of scrofula ?

Even when a material substance, applied to the skin, or introduced into a wound, has propagated disease by infection,

---

* Life was suddenly endangered by injecting a little pure water into a vein. *See Mullen, in Birch, History of the Royal Society,* vol. iv.

Atmospheric air introduced into the veins has occasioned death. *See J. H. Voigt, Magazin für den neusten Zustand der Naturkunde,* vol. i. iii. p. 25.

Even the mildest liquids, introduced into the veins, have placed life in danger. *See Autenrieth, Physiologie,* ii. § 784.

who can prove (what has so often been affirmed in our Pa-
thogeny) that the slightest particle of this material substance
penetrates into our liquids or becomes absorbed?* It is in
vain to wash the genitals with care and promptitude, such
precaution will not protect the system from the venereal virus.
The least breath of air emanating from a patient labouring
under small-pox is sufficient to produce that formidable disease
in a healthy child.

How much of this material principle—what quantity in
weight—would be requisite for the liquids to imbibe, in order
to produce, in the first instance, syphilis, which will continue
during the whole term of life ; and, in the second, the small-
pox, which often rapidly destroys life amidst a suppuration †
almost general ?

Is it possible in these two cases, or in others which are
analogous, to admit that a morbific principle, in a material
form, could have introduced itself into the blood? It has

---

* A young girl, of Glasgow, eight years of age, having been bitten by a
mad dog, the surgeon *immediately cut out the part*, which, nevertheless, did
not save the child from an attack of hydrophobia thirty-six days after, of
which she died at the end of two days. *Med. Comment. of Edinb. Dec.* 2,
vol. ii. 1793.

† In order to account for the great quantity of putrid fœcal matter, and
fetid ichorous discharge, which arises in disease, and to represent these substances as the cause that calls forth, and keeps up, the morbid state, although,
at the moment of infection, nothing material had been seen to enter into the
body, they had recourse to another hypothesis, which admitted, that certain
very minute contagious principles act upon the body as a ferment, bringing the
humours into the same degree of corruption with themselves, and converting
them in this manner into a similar ferment, which keeps up the disease. But,
by what purifying decoctions do they expect to free the body from a ferment
that is constantly renewed, and expel it so completely from the mass of
fluids, that not a single particle may remain, which, according to the admitted
hypothesis, if any did remain, would infallibly corrupt the humours afresh, and
reproduce, as at first, new morbific principles? Thus, according to the
manner of the old school, it would be impossible ever to cure these diseases.
Here we see to what absurd conclusions the most artful hypothesis will lead,
if founded in error. The most firmly rooted syphilis, when the psoric affection with which it is often complicated, has been removed, may be cured by
one or two small doses of a solution of mercury, diluted to the decillionth
potence, whereby the general syphilitic corruption of the humours is (dynamically) corrected in a permanent and constitutional manner.

often happened that a letter, written in the chamber of a patient, has communicated the same contagious disease to the person who read it. Can we entertain the opinion, that any thing material entered into the humours in this instance? But why all these proofs? How often have we seen that an offensive or vexatious word has brought on a bilious fever which endangered life ;—a superstitious prophecy of death, actually occasion death at the very epoch predicted; afflicting news, or an agreeable surprise, suddenly suspend the vital powers! Where is there, in any of these cases, the morbific material principle which entered, in substance, into the body, which produced disease and kept it up, and, without the expulsion or destruction of which, by medicines, all radical cure would be impossible?

The supporters of an hypothesis so gross as that of morbific principles, ought to blush, that they have so thoughtlessly overlooked and disregarded the spiritual nature of our life, and the spiritual dynamic power of morbific agents, and have thus reduced themselves to mere scouring physicians, who, instead of curing, destroy life, by their attempts to drive out of the body peccant matters which never had an existence there.

In diseases, the excretions which are often so disgusting, could they be the actual material which produced the malady, and which kept it up?* Are they not rather *the product of the disease itself; that is to say, of the pure dynamic derangement which the constitution has undergone?*

With such erroneous ideas of the material origin and essence of disease, it is by no means surprising, that, in all ages, the obscure as well as the distinguished practitioner, together with the inventors of the most sublime theories, should have for their principal aim, the separation and expulsion of a supposed morbid material, and that the indication most frequently established, was that of dividing this material, rendering it movable, and expelling it by the saliva, the bronchial mucus, the urine, and perspiration; purifying the blood by the action

---

* If this were true, it would be sufficient to blow the nose, and wipe it clean, to effect a speedy and infallible cure of all species of coryza, even the most inveterate.

of herbal decoctions, (which are supposed to effect this process at the command of the physician,) thus unloading it of acrid matter and impurities which it *never contained;* drawing off the imaginary principle of the disease mechanically, by means of setons, cauteries, permanent blisters; and above all, by the expulsion of the peccant matter, as they termed it, through the intestinal canal, by laxatives and purgatives; and, to add to their importance, they were dignified with the high-sounding titles of *aperients and dissolvents.* All of these were so many attempts to remove a hostile material principle which never did and never could have existed.

Now, if we admit that—which is an established fact—namely, that with the exception of those diseases brought on by the introduction of indigestible or hurtful substances into the alimentary canal and other organs,—those produced by foreign bodies penetrating the skin, &c.,—there does not exist a single disease that can have a material principle for its cause. On the contrary, all of them are solely and always the special result of an actual and dynamic derangement in the state of health; how contradictory, then, must that method of treatment, which depends upon the expulsion* of this

---

* There is, apparently, some necessity for the expulsion of worms in the so-called worm-disease. But even this appearance is false. A few *lumbrici* are found in some children, and *ascarides* in a greater number. But the greater part of either one or the other is owing to a general affection (psoric) connected with an unhealthy mode of living. If the regimen be ameliorated, and the psoric affection homœopathically cured, which is easier to be performed at this age than at any other period of life, there will remain but few or no worms at all, or at least, the children are no longer incommoded by them; whereas, on the other hand, they promptly appear again, in great numbers, after the administration of mere purgatives, even combined with wormseed. "But the tape-worm, this monster, created for the torment of human nature, *must* certainly be driven out with all manner of force." Yes, *at times,* he will be driven out, but beneath what sufferings and danger! I should not like to have upon my conscience the death of all those who have fallen sacrifices to the violence of purgatives directed against this worm, or the long years of debility which they, who escaped death, must have dragged out. And how often does it not occur, that after having repeated these purgatives, so destructive to life and health, during several years successively, the animal is either not driven out at all, or is re-produced! How then, if there be no necessity at all for seeking to expel and destroy the tænia by means so violent and cruel, and which place the life of the patient in such

imaginary principle, appear to every reasonable man, since no good can result from it, in treating the principal diseases of mankind, viz., the chronic, but, on the contrary, much mischief!

No one will deny, that the degenerate and impure substances which appear in diseases, are anything else than the mere product of disease itself, which the system can get rid of, in a forcible manner, frequently too forcible, without the aid of evacuating medicines, and that they are reproduced so long as the disease continues. These substances often appear, to the true physician, in the shape of morbid symptoms, and aid him in discovering the nature and image of the disease, which he afterwards avails himself of, in performing a cure by means of homœopathic agents.

————

imminent danger! The different species of tænia are only found in patients labouring under a psoric affection; and when the latter is cured, they instantly disappear. Until the cure is accomplished, they live, without being a source of great inconvenience to the patient, not exactly in the intestines, but amid the residue of the aliments, where they exist without doing injury, and find what they require for their nourishment. As long as this state of things continues, they do not touch the coats of the intestines, or do any harm to the body that contains them; but the first moment that an acute disease attacks the patient, the contents of the intestines become insupportable to the animal, which turns itself about and irritates the sensitive part of the entrails, exciting a species of spasmodic colic, which adds greatly to the sufferings of the invalid. In the same manner, the child is restless, turns and pushes, while the mother is sick, but floats quietly in the amniotic fluid, without inconvenience to her, when she is well. It may be observed here, that the symptoms which manifest themselves at this epoch, with persons who have the solitary worm within them, are of such a nature, that often the smallest dose of tincture of male-fern-root (*filex* mas.) speedily effects their eradication in a homœopathic manner, because it puts an end to that part of the malady occasioned by the disturbed state of the animal: the tape-worm, finding itself once more at ease, continues to exist upon the intestinal substances, without incommoding the patient in any very painful degree, until the anti-psoric cure is so far advanced that the worm no longer finds the contents of the intestinal canal fit for his support, and he voluntarily quits it forever, without any purgatives being employed.

But the most skilful among the present followers of the
former school of medicine do not wish it to be known, that the
chief aim of their mode of treatment, is the expulsion of material morbid principles. To the numerous evacuants which
they employ, they apply the name of *derivatives*, and in so doing, pretend that they do nothing more than imitate the nature of the disordered system, which, in her efforts to re-estab-
lish health, distinguishes fever by sweats and urine ; pleurisy
by bleedings at the nose, perspiration, and mucous expectoration ; other diseases by vomiting, diarrhœa, and hemorrhoidal
flux ; articular pains, by ulcers on the legs ; angina by salivation, &c., or by metastasis and abscesses which she forms in
parts distant from the seat of the disease.

Accordingly, they think they can do nothing better than
imitate nature, and thus they adopt an indirect mode of treatment in the majority of diseases. They follow the traces of
the diseased vital power left to itself, and proceed in an indirect manner,* by applying stronger heterogeneous irritation
to parts distant from the seat of the disease, exciting and
keeping up evacuations by the organs dissimilar to the tissues
affected, in order to turn the course of the evil, in some degree, towards this new position.

*This derivative system was, and still continues, one of the
chief curative indications of the prevailing school.*

By this imitation of self-helping nature, *vis medicatrix
naturæ*, as it is termed by others, they try to excite, by forcible
means, (in the parts least affected, and which can best support the malady which the medicines provoke,) fresh symptoms which extinguish the primitive disease,† by assuming
the appearance of a crisis, and thus allow the powers of self-
helping nature to operate a gradual resolution.‡

* Instead of extinguishing the evil promptly, and without delay, as in the
homœopathic mode of treatment, by the application of dynamic medicinal
powers, directed against the diseased parts of the system.

† As if anything immaterial could be drawn off! Yet they suppose a
morbid material, be it as subtle as it may.

‡ Diseases that are moderately acute, are the only ones that terminate
quietly, when they have reached the natural term of their career, whether
weak allœopathic remedies be applied to them or otherwise : the vital powers,
when reviving, gradually substitute the normal state in the place of the in-

They recommend diaphoretics, diuretics, venesection, setons, and cauteries, and above all, excite irritation of the alimentary canal, so as to produce evacuations from above, and more especially from below, all of which were irritatives, and to these they applied the names of aperients and dissolvents.*

In aid of this derivative system they likewise employ another which bears great affinity to it, and which consists of *counter-irritants:* lamb's wool applied to the bare skin, footbaths, nauseants, the cure by infliction of the torments of hunger upon the intestinal canal, (abstinence,) applications that excite pains, inflammation, and suppuration in the neighbouring or distant parts, such as, armoracia, sinapisms, blisters, mezereum, the seton, Autenrieth's ointment, (ointment of emetic tartar,) the moxa, actual cautery, the acupuncture, &c. And in this, they again follow the example of pure nature, which, left to herself, endeavours to get rid of the dynamic disease by pains, which she causes to arise in the distant regions of the body, by metastasis and abscesses; by cutaneous eruptions or suppurating ulcers; but all her efforts, in this respect, are useless, where the disease is of a chronic nature.

Thus it is evident, that it was no well-digested plan, but merely *imitation*, that led the old school to these helpless, pernicious, and indirect methods of cure, both derivative and counter-irritant; and induced them to adopt plans of treatment so inefficacious, debilitating, and injurious, in ameliorating and dissipating disease, which arouse another and worse evil to occupy the place of the former. Can we call that healing which rather deserves to be called destroying? for the name of cure could never be applied to such a result. They were contented to follow nature in the efforts which

---

normal. But in every acute disease, and in those that are chronic, which constitute the great majority of diseases to which man is subject, this resource no longer comes to the aid of simple nature, and the old school of medicine. The efforts of the vital powers, and the imitative attempts of allœopathy, are not potent enough to effect a resolution; and all that results from them is a truce of short duration, during which the enemy gathers his forces to re-appear, sooner or later, in a more formidable shape than ever.

* This very denomination likewise announces a supposition on their part of the presence of some morbific substance which was to be dissolved and expelled.

4

she makes, and which are only crowned with partial success[*] in acute diseases of a mild form.

They did nothing more than imitate the preserving vital

* The ordinary school of medicine regarded the means which the organism employs to relieve itself, in those patients who make no use of medicines, as perfect models of imitation ; but they were *greatly mistaken*. The miserable and very imperfect attempts which the vital powers make to assist themselves in acute diseases, is a spectacle that ought to excite man to use all the resources of his learning and wisdom, to put an end, by a real cure, to this torment, which nature herself inflicts. If nature cannot cure, homœopathically, a disease already existing in the system, by the production of a fresh malady *similar* to it, (sec. 43—46,) a thing not often in her power to effect, (sec. 50,) and if the system, deprived of all external succour, stands alone to triumph over a malady that has just broken out, (her resistance is totally powerless in chronic miasms,) we see nothing but painful and often dangerous efforts of the constitution to save itself at all hazards, efforts of which death is most frequently the result.

Just as little as we can witness what is passing in the interior of our bodies in a healthy condition, and as certainly as these processes remain concealed from us, as they lie open to the sight of Omniscience—just so little can we perceive the internal operations of the animal frame, when life is disturbed by disease. The action that takes place in diseases manifests itself only by external symptoms, through the medium of which alone our system expresses the troubles that take place in the interior ; so that, in each given case, we never once discover which are those among the morbid symptoms that owe their origin to the primitive action of the disease, and those which are occasioned by the re-action of the vital powers endeavouring to rescue themselves from danger. Both are confounded before our eyes, and only present to us, (reflected on the exterior,) an image of the entire malady within ; since the fruitless efforts by which nature, abandoned to herself, makes, to put an end to the malady, are also sufferings which the whole frame undergoes. This is the reason why those evacuations which nature usually excites at the termination of diseases, that have been rapid in their attacks, and which are called crises, often do more harm than good. What the vital powers do in these pretended crises, and in what manner they are accomplished, are mysteries to us, as well as every other internal action which takes place in the organic economy of life. One thing, however, is certain, which is, that in the course of these efforts, there are particular parts that suffer *more or less, and which are sacrificed to the safety of others*. These operations of the vital power proceeding to combat an acute disease, solely in conformity to the laws of the organic constitution, and not according to the inspirations of a reflecting mind, are, for the most part, merely a section of allœopathy. In order to free the organs primitively affected, by means of a crisis, it increases the activity of the organs of secretion in order to lead off the evil from the former to the latter : thence result vomiting,

powers abandoned to their own resources, which, depending
solely upon the organic laws of the body, only act in virtue of
these laws, without reasoning or reflecting upon their actions.
They copied nature, who could not, like an intelligent surgeon,
bring together the gaping lips of a wound, and reunite them
by the first intention; who, in an oblique fracture, can do
nothing, however great may be the quantity of osseous matter
which exudes, to adjust and attach the two ends of the bone;
who, not knowing how to tie up a wounded artery, suffers a
man full of strength and health to bleed to death; who, ignorant of the art of reducing a dislocation, renders its reduction
in a very short time impossible, by reason of the swelling
which she excites in all the neighbouring parts; who, in order
to free herself from a foreign body that had penetrated the
transparent cornea, destroys the whole eye by suppuration;
who, in a strangulated hernia, cannot break the obstacle but
by gangrene and death; who, finally, in dynamic diseases, by
changing their form, often renders the state of the patient worse
than it was before. Besides, *this unintelligent vital power admits into the body, without hesitation*, the greatest scourge of our
earthly existence, the source of countless diseases which have
afflicted the human species for centuries past—that is to say,
chronic miasms, such as psora, syphilis, and sycosis. And, far
from being able to relieve the system of any one of these
miasms, she does not even possess the power of ameliorating
them; but, on the contrary, suffers them quietly to continue

diarrhœa, plentiful flow of urine, sweats, abscesses, &c.; and the nervous
powers, attacked dynamically, seek, in some degree, to unload themselves by
material products.

The animal economy, abandoned to its own resources, cannot save itself
from acute diseases, but by the destruction and sacrifice of one part of the
system itself; and even where death does not ensue, the harmony of life and
health is restored only in a slow and imperfect manner.

The great debility of those organs which have been exposed to the attacks
of the malady, as well as that of the entire body, after this spontaneous cure,
meagreness, &c., are sufficient testimonies of the truth of what we have asserted.

In short, the whole proceedings by which the system delivers itself from
the diseases with which it is attacked, only exhibit to the observer a tissue
of sufferings, and show him nothing which he can or ought to imitate, if he
truly exercises the art of healing.

their ravages until death comes to close the eyes of the patient, after long years of grief and suffering.

In a matter so important as that of healing,—in a profession that requires so much intelligence, judgment, and skill,—how could the old school (which was accounted rational) blindly take the vital power for its best instructor and guide ; how could it venture, without reflection, to imitate the indirect and revolutionary acts which the vital power performs in disease— and, finally, follow it as the best and most perfect of models, whilst reason, that magnificent gift of the Deity, has been granted to us, in order that we may go infinitely beyond it, in the aid which we are to bring to our fellow mortals ?

When the prevailing school of medicine, in the accustomed application of their repellent and derivative systems of cure, (which have no other basis than an inconsiderate imitation of the natural, automatic powers of life,) attack the healthy organs, and inflict on them pains more acute than those of the disease itself against which they are directed—or, what happens more frequently, force evacuations, which dissipate in pure loss the strength and the juices ;—their aim is to direct towards the parts which they irritate, that morbid action which life developed in the organs that were primitively affected, and thus violently uproot the natural disease, *by exciting a stronger heterogeneous disease* in the more healthy parts—that is to say, by making use of indirect and circuitous means, which exhaust the powers and occasion great suffering.*

* Daily experience shows us how unsuccessful these manœuvres are in chronic diseases. *In very few cases is a cure effected.* But can they call that a victory, where instead of attacking the enemy in front, hand to hand, and terminating the difference by his death, they content themselves with setting every part of the country behind him in flames, cutting off retreat and destroying all around. By such means they may certainly succeed in breaking the courage of their adversary, but their object is still unattained ; the foe is not destroyed, he is still there ; and when his magazines are replenished, he again rears his head, more ferocious than he was before.—The enemy, I say, is not destroyed, but the poor innocent country is so ruined that it will scarce recover itself in a long lapse of time. This is precisely what happens to allœopathy, in chronic diseases, when, without curing the malady, it undermines and destroys the system by indirect attacks against innocent organs, which are distant from the seat of the latter. These are the results of such injurious attempts.

It is true, that by these heterogeneous attacks, the disease, when it is an acute one, (and consequently cannot be of long duration,) transports itself to parts distant and dissimilar to those which it at first occupied; but it is by no means cured. There is nothing in this revolutionary mode of treatment that has a direct or immediate connection with the organs primitively diseased, or which deserves to be called *a cure*. By abstaining from such grievous attacks upon the life of the other parts of the system, the acute disease would often dissipate itself even more rapidly, leaving less suffering behind, and without occasioning so great a consumption of the powers. Besides, neither the mode of proceeding which is followed by simple nature, nor its allœopathic imitation, will bear a comparison with the direct, dynamic, homœopathic treatment, which, without wasting the vital powers, extinguishes the disease in a prompt and rapid manner.

But in the great majority of diseases, and in chronic affections, these stormy, debilitating, and indirect treatments of the old school scarcely ever produce any good. All that they can effect is, a suspension, for a few days, of some incommodious symptom or another, which returns immediately, when nature has become accustomed to the distant irritation; the disease then returns more grievous than before, because the repellant pains* and the ill-advised evacuations have lessened the energy of the vital powers.

While the greater number of allœopathic physicians, in their *general imitation* of the salutary effects of nature, abandoned to her own resources, thus introduced into the practice of medicine those derivative systems which they termed useful, and which every one varied according to the fancied indications suggested by his own ideas; others, aiming at a still higher

* What favourable consequences have ever resulted from issues, so frequently established, diffusing their fetid odours around? Even though they appear during the first fortnight, by their irritating power, slightly to diminish a chronic disease as long as they continue to keep up considerable pain, they afterwards, when the body is accustomed to the pain, have *no other* effect than that of weakening the patient, and thus opening a still wider field to the chronic affection. Or, are there yet physicians in the nineteenth century who could regard these issues as outlets for the escape of the peccant matters? It appears that some such practitioners do exist!

object, promoted with all their skill the tendency which the
vital powers *exhibit in diseases, to relieve themselves by evacuations, and opposing metastasis, and endeavoured in some degree
to aid them,* by promoting these derivations and evacuations,
imagining that by this mode of treatment they might justly
arrogate to themselves the names *ministri naturæ.* Because it
often happens, in chronic diseases, that the evacuations which
nature excites, bring relief in cases where there are acute pains,
paralysis, spasms, &c., the old school imagined that the true
method of curing disease was by favouring, keeping up, or
even increasing the evacuations. But they never discovered
that all those pretended crises, those evacuations and derivations produced by nature abandoned to her own exertions, only
procure palliative relief for a short period, and that, far from
contributing towards a real cure, they, on the contrary, aggravate the internal primitive evil, by consuming the strength and
the juices. No one has ever seen those efforts of simple nature
effect the durable recovery of a patient, nor have those evacuations, excited by the system,* ever cured a chronic disease.
On the contrary, in all cases of this nature, after a short relief,
(the duration of which gradually diminishes,) the primitive
affection is manifestly aggravated, and the attacks return
stronger and more frequent than before, although the evacuations do not cease.

In the same manner, nature, abandoned to her own resources
in internal chronic diseases which threaten life, can only bring
relief by exciting the appearance of external local symptoms,
in order to turn away danger from the organs indispensable to
existence, and transport it, by metastasis, to those which are
not so; such attempts of an unintelligent, inconsiderate but
energetic vital force, have a tendency towards anything but a
real cure ; they are nothing more than palliatives, short stag-
nations imposed on the internal disease, at the sacrifice of a
great portion of the liquids and strength, without the primitive
affection losing anything of its intensity. Without the aid of
homœopathic treatment, all they can do, at farthest, is to
delay for a time that death which is inevitable.

The Allœopathy of the old school greatly exaggerated the

* Not more effectual are those artificially produced.

efforts of pure nature. Falsely judging them to be truly salutary, they sought to promote and develop them still farther,
hoping, by these means, to destroy the entire evil and effect a
radical cure. When, in a chronic disease, the vital power
appeared to improve this or that grievous symptom of the internal state, for example, by means of a humid exanthema, then
the self-styled minister of nature applied a blister, or some other
exutory, upon the suppurating surface, to draw (*duce natura*)
a still greater quantity of humour from the skin, and thus assist
nature in the cure, by removing from the body the morbific
principle. But sometimes, when the action of the remedy was
too violent, the humid tetter already old, and the body too susceptible of irritation, the external affection increased considerably, without any advantage accruing to the primitive evil; and
the pains, rendered still more acute, deprived the patient of
sleep, diminished his strength, and often brought on a bad description of feverish erysipelas. Sometimes, when the remedy
acted with more gentleness upon the local disease, (which was
perhaps yet recent,) it exercised a kind of external homœopathy
upon the local symptoms which nature had produced upon the
skin, in order to relieve the internal malady; thus renewing the
latter, to which still greater danger was attached, and exposing
the vital powers by the suppression of the local symptoms, to
the excitement of others of a graver nature, in other and more
noble parts. The patient then was attacked with a dangerous
ophthalmy, deafness, spasms in the stomach, epileptic convulsions, suffocation, fits of apoplexy, mental derangement, &c.*
The same pretext of assisting the vital powers in their curative efforts, led the minister of nature, when the malady caused
an afflux of blood into the veins of the rectum, or the anus,
(blind piles,) to have recourse to the repeated application of
leeches in great numbers, in order to open an issue to the
blood in that quarter. The emission of blood procured an
amendment, sometimes so slight, as to be scarce deserving of
notice; but, at the same time, it weakened the body and gave

* These are the natural results of repelling such local symptoms—results,
which the allœopathic physician often regards as diseases that are perfectly
new and of a different character.

rise to a yet stronger congestion towards the extremity of the intestinal canal, without effecting the slightest diminution of the primitive malady.

In almost every case, where the diseased vital powers endeavoured to evacuate a little blood by vomiting, expectoration, &c., in order to diminish the severity of a dangerous internal affection, they immediately hastened (*duce natura*) to give all the assistance in their power to these pretended salutary efforts of nature, and blood in abundance was extracted from the vein ; which never failed to prove injurious in the end, and to weaken the body to a manifest extent.

And still more frequently, with the intent of assisting nature, in chronic nausea, they excited powerful evacuations of the stomach and administered plentiful emetics ; but never with any good result, and seldom without frightful and even dangerous consequences. To appease the internal malady in a slight degree, the vital powers sometimes excite indolent enlargements of the external glands. The minister of nature thinks he is serving the divinity to whom he is devoted, by bringing these tumours to a suppuration, by the use of frictions and warm applications, in order to plunge the knife into the abscess when it is arrived at maturity, and cause the peccant matter to flow externally.(?) But experience has a thousand times proved the interminable evils that always result from this mode of treatment.

Because the allœopathist has often seen severe sufferings, in chronic diseases, somewhat relieved by spontaneous nocturnal perspiration, or by certain natural dejections of liquid matter, he thinks himself bound to follow these indications of nature ; he likewise thinks it his duty to second the labours which he sees carried on in his own presence, by prescribing a complete sudorific treatment, or the continued use, during several years, of what he calls gentle laxatives, in order to relieve the patient of the disease that torments him with more speed and certainty. But this mode of treatment never produces anything but a contrary result, that is to say, it always aggravates the primitive disease.

Thus the allœopathist, yielding to the force of this opinion, which he has embraced without scrutiny, notwithstanding the absence of all foundation, persists in seconding* the efforts of the diseased vital powers, and augmenting the derivations and evacuations, which never lead to the attainment of his object, but rather to the ruin of the patient. He never discovers that local affections, evacuations, and apparent derivations, (which are effects excited and kept up by the vital powers abandoned to their own resources, in order to afford some slight relief to the primitive disease,) are of themselves a constituent part of the *ensemble* of the signs of the malady, against the totality of which there could be no real, salutary, and curative remedy, save a medicine whose effects were analogous with the phenomena occasioned by its action upon man when in a state of health, or, in other terms, a homœopathic remedy.

As every thing that simple nature performs to relieve herself in acute, and more particularly, in chronic diseases, is highly imperfect, and is actually *disease itself*, it may readily be conceived that the efforts of art labouring to assist this imperfection do still greater injury; and in acute maladies, at least, they cannot remedy that which is defective in the attempts of nature, because the physician, incapable of following the concealed paths by which the vital power accomplishes its crisis, could only operate upon the exterior by means of energetic remedies, whose effects not only do less

* The old school, however, often permitted themselves to follow an inverse method of treatment: that is, when the efforts of nature, tending to relieve the internal malady by evacuations, or by exciting local external symptoms, manifestly injured the patient, they employ against them all the powers of repellents; and thus combat chronic pains, insomnolency, and diarrhœa of long standing, with strong and hazardous doses of opium; vomitings, by effervescing mixtures; fœtid perspiration of the feet, by cold foot-baths and astringent fomentations; eruptions of the skin, with preparations of lead and zinc; uterine hemorrhages, by injections of vinegar; colliquative perspirations, by alum curd; nocturnal seminal emissions, by the use of camphor in large quantities; sudden glow of heat over the face and body, by nitric, sulphuric, and vegetable acids; bleedings at the nostrils, with dossils of lint dipped in alcohol or astringent liquids; ulcers on the lower extremities, by oxides of lead, zinc, &c. But thousands of facts attest the melancholy consequences that result from this mode of treatment. The allœopathist, both in speaking and writing, boasts of being a rational physician, of searching out the latent cause of disease, and always of effecting radical cures; but it is evident that a treatment founded on isolated symptoms must always be detrimental to the patient.

good than those of nature, abandoned to herself, but on the
contrary, are more perturbating and destructive to the powers.
Even this imperfect relief, which nature effects by means of
derivations and crises, he cannot attain by following the same
path ; do what he will, even the miserable succour which the
vital powers can procure, when abandoned to their own resources, is infinitely beyond the skill of the allœopathist.

By a scarification of the pituitary membrane, it has been
tried to produce bleeding at the nose, in imitation of natural
nasal hemorrhage, to relieve, for example, an attack of chronic cephalalgy. In such a case, a quantity of blood might be
drawn from the nostrils sufficient to weaken the patient ; but
the relief would be far less than that afforded at another time
when the vital instinctive powers, of their own accord, caused
only a few drops of blood to flow.

One of those so-called critical perspirations or diarrhœas,
which the incessant activity of the vital powers excites, after
any sudden indisposition arising from vexation, fright, cold, or
injury from improper lifting, is far more efficacious in allaying,
momentarily at least, the acute suffering of the patient, than
all the nauseous sudorifics or purgatives contained in the
shop of an apothecary. This is proved beyond a doubt by
daily experience.

However, the vital power, which is devoid of intelligence
and judgment, and which cannot act of itself, but according
to the organic disposition of our bodies, was not given to us
that we should follow it as our best guide in the cure of diseases, much less that we should imitate, in a servile manner,
its imperfect attempts to restore health by joining to it a treatment more opposed than its own to the object it has in view,
for no other purpose than that of sparing ourselves the study
and reflection necessary to the discovery of the true art of
healing, and finally to place a bad copy of the inefficacious
aid which nature affords when abandoned to her own resources, in the room of the most noble of all human arts !
What reflecting man would copy the efforts of nature in curing disease ? These very efforts are the disease itself, and
the morbidly affected vital energy is evidently the source of
the malady. It follows, then, that to imitate or to suppress
these efforts must in one case augment them, or in the other

render them dangerous by suppression, and the allœopathist does both ; these are their pernicious doings, who boast of following the rational plan of healing !

No ; that innate power of man which directs life in the most perfect manner *whilst in health*, whose presence is alike felt in every part of the system, in the sensitive as in the irritable fibre, and which is the indefatigable spring of all the normal functions of the body, was not created for the purpose of aiding itself in disease. *It does not exercise a system of cure that is worthy of imitation, that is to say, a work of reflection and judgment, and which, when the automatic and unintelligent vital powers have been disordered by disease, and in-normal action produced, knows how to modify them by appropriate remedies, so that after the disappearance of the new disease produced by the medicine, (which soon takes place,) they return to their normal state, and to their appointed function of maintaining health in the system, without having undergone, during this conversion, any painful or debilitating attacks.   Homœopathic medicine teaches us the mode by which we are to arrive at this result.*

———

A great number of patients treated according to the methods of the old school, which have just passed in review before us, escaped from diseases, not in chronic disorders, (non-venereal,) but in those maladies that were acute, and which are less dangerous. This, however, was effected by such painfully circuitous means, and frequently in a manner so imperfect, that no one could say the cure was performed by the influence of an art that acted mildly in its mode of treatment. In cases where there was no imminent danger, acute diseases were sometimes repressed by means of venesection, or sometimes by the suppression of one of the principal symptoms, by a palliative enantiopathic remedy, (*contraria contrariis*), or sometimes suspended by irritants and revulsants applied to parts removed from the diseased organ, until the course of their natural revolution was ended—that is to say, they opposed them by indirect means, exhausting the strength and

the juices; so that the greater part of what was necessary
to be done, in order to remove the disease and repair the losses
which the patient had undergone, remained to be performed
by the self-preserving vital power. The latter, then, had not
only to subdue the acute natural disease, but also to overcome
the results of an ill-directed mode of treatment. In casual
cases, this vital power was to exercise its own energies
to bring back the functions to their normal rhythm, which
could only be effected imperfectly and slowly, and with great
difficulty.

In acute diseases, it is doubtful whether this treatment of
the existing school really facilitates or abridges the cure by
the aid of nature, since neither of them act but in an indirect
manner; and their derivative and counter-irritating modes of
cure, wound the system more profoundly, and lead to a still
greater dissipation of the vital powers.

———

The old school practise yet another method of cure, which
they call " exciting and strengthening,"* (by *excitantia, nervina, tonica, confortantia, roborantia*.) It is surprising that they
should boast of this mode of treatment.

Has it ever succeeded in removing the weakness which a
chronic disease so often engenders, augments, and keeps up,
by prescribing (as it has so frequently done) etheric Rhine
wine, or spirituous Tokay? As this treatment was not able
to cure the chronic disease, (the source of the debility,) the
strength of the patient decreased in proportion as they made
him take more wine, because the vital powers, in their reaction, oppose relaxation to artificial excitements.

Did cinchona, or any of the mistaken, ambiguous and pernicious substances, which collectively bear the name of *Amara*, ever restore strength in these cases which are of such frequent occurrence? These vegetable products, which they

* This method is, properly speaking, enantiopathic, and I will again touch
upon it in the course of the Organon, (sec. 59.)

pretended were tonic and strengthening in all circumstances,
together with the preparations of iron, did they not add fresh
sufferings to the old ones, by reason of their peculiar morbific
action, without being able to remove the debility which depended on an unknown malady of long standing?

The so-called *unguenta nervina*, or the other spirituous and
balsamic topical applications, did they ever diminish in a durable manner, or even momentarily, incipient paralysis of an
arm or leg, (which arises, as is frequently the case, from a
chronic disease,) without curing the cause itself? Or have
electric and galvanic shocks ever produced, in such cases, any
other results than those of gradually increasing the paralysis
of the muscular irritability and the nervous* susceptibility,
and finally rendering the paralysis complete?

Have not the highly-boasted *excitantia* and *aphrodisiaca*,
ambergris, smelts, tincture of cantharides, truffles, cardamoms,
cinnamon, and vanilla, constantly ended with changing the
gradually declining power of the virile faculties (which is always caused by some unobserved chronic miasm) into total
impotence?

How could they boast of an acquisition of strength, and excitement, which lasts only a few hours, when the results that
follow bring on an opposite state (which is lasting) according
to the laws of all palliatives?

The little good that the *excitantia* and *roborantia* did to the
patient treated for acute maladies, according to the old method, was a thousand times overbalanced by the ill effects which
the use of them produced in chronic diseases.

The allœopathists not unfrequently commence the treatment of a chronic disease by blindly administering their so-
called alterative remedies, (*alterantia*,) among which the
mercurials (calomel, blue pill, corrosive sublimate, mercurial
ointments) occupy a conspicuous place. These sovereign

---

* An apothecary (in Jever) had a voltaic column, the gradual strokes of
which gave temporary relief to persons afflicted with deafness. Soon these
shocks caused no more effect, and it was necessary, in order to produce the
same results, to render them yet stronger, until, in their turn, they likewise
became inefficacious: after this, the most powerful shocks only had the faculty, at the commencement, of restoring the hearing of the patient for a few
hours, but finished by leaving him a prey to total deafness.

remedies of theirs, even in cases not venereal, are often given
in large and long-continued doses, until their deleterious tendency becomes manifest in the ruined health of the patient.
Great alterations are certainly produced by the destructive
operation of mercury upon improper parts, but they are such
as finally exhaust the constitution of the patient.

Cinchona, in all genuine marsh intermittents, is a homœopathic remedy, and when not prevented by pre-existing psora,
a specific. But by prescribing it in large and long-continued
doses in every epidemic intermittent, the ignorance of the old
school is abundantly shown; for, the disease almost every
year assuming a different character, requires for its removal a
different homœopathic remedy, which in a single dose, or, at
most, a very few minute doses, effects a radical cure in the
course of a few days. Now, because such epidemic fevers
have their periodical attacks, (type of the disease,) while it is
these which an allœopathist chiefly regards in an intermittent,
and while the bark is considered as the only remedy for its removal, if he can but suppress the type of the disease by means
of enormous doses of that medicine, or its more costly extract,
quinine, he supposes, forsooth, that the patient is cured. But
he is really left in a worse condition after such suppression of
the periodical returns of his fever, than before. We behold
him moving slowly along, his countenance sallow, his breathing asthmatic, the hypochondres distended, the abdominal
viscera diseased, frequently the abdomen itself and limbs in a
bloated condition,—without healthful appetite or refreshing
sleep, weak and dispirited, he is discharged from the hospital
in this state of complicated suffering—as cured! not unfrequently years of elaborate homœopathic treatment are required, we will not say to restore his health, but to rescue this
radically vitiated, this artificially cachectic patient from an
untimely death.

It is cause of gratification to the old school when, by the
antipathic virtues of *valerian*, they can convert the stupor of
nervous fever into a degree of exhilaration for a few hours.
But this transient excitement being once over, it can be reproduced only by a repetition of still larger doses of the same
medicine, and even the largest soon lose their effect. Their
primary operation being that of a stimulating palliative, the

entire vital energies, during the secondary effects of the medicine, become paralyzed, and thus, by means of the *rational* treatment of the old school, the speedy dissolution of the patient is rendered inevitable. As certainly mortal as is the issue of the case, the followers of the old system do not perceive it, and the patient's death is ascribed by them to the malignity of his disease.

Digitalis purpurea is a still more formidable palliative in chronic diseases, and its virtues are highly extolled by the old school for allaying the rapid and irritated pulse (purely symptomatic) in these maladies. Though the use of this potent enantiopathic medicine may at first, in many instances, abate the frequency of the pulse for some hours, yet it will shortly afterwards become more frequent than ever. To retard its velocity again, the medicine is repeated in a larger dose ; it is again availing, yet for a shorter period ; until by frequent repetition, even in augmented doses, it loses its effects altogether. The pulse not now being restrained by the secondary or consecutive effects of digitalis, becomes more rampant than before its use, and too rapid to be reckoned. Among the train of consequences may also be observed, loss of sleep and appetite and diminution of strength, until, finally, if these disasters do not terminate in incurable mania, death becomes the patient's only refuge !*

Such, then, was the treatment which the allœopathic physician practised on his patients. The latter, therefore, were obliged to yield to necessity, since they could derive nothing better from the other physicians who had drawn their information from the same fallacious source.

The fundamental cause of chronic diseases, (non venereal,) and the mode by which they could be cured, remained unknown to these practitioners, who prided themselves on their own remedies, which they said were directed against the

---

* Notwithstanding all this, Hufeland, the representative of the old school, with great self-complacency, in his pamphlet on homœopathia, p. 22, praises the *digitalis* for the purpose of repressing morbid frequency of the pulse : his words are, " None will deny " (but experience does) " that a too vehement circulation can be removed by digitalis " (?) permanently ? does he mean *removed ?* what ! by the use of an heroic enantiopathic remedy ? Poor Hufeland !

cause. How was it possible for them to cure the immense
number of chronic diseases by their indirect methods, their imperfect imitations of the efforts of an automatic vital power,
which were never destined to become models of a treatment
to be followed in medicine ?

They regarded that which they believed to be the character
of the malady, as the cause of the disease itself, and, accordingly, directed their pretended radical cures against spasm,
inflammation, (plethora,) fever, general or partial debility,
pituita, putridity, obstructions, &c., which they imagined they
could remove with the aid of their antispasmodics, antiphlogistics, tonics, irritants, antiseptics, dissolvents, resolutives,
derivatives, evacuants, and other repellent medicines, known
to themselves only in a superficial manner.

But indications of so vague a nature were insufficient to
discover those medicines which are of real utility, particularly
so in the materia medica of the old school, which, as I have
elsewhere shown,* depended mostly upon mere conjecture,
and on false conclusions *ab usu in morbis*, mixed up with fraud
and falsehood.

They continued to act with the same degree of coldness in
matters that were still more hypothetical; against the deficiency or superabundance of oxygen, nitrogen, carbon, and
hydrogen, in the fluids; against the exaltation or diminution of
irritability, sensibility, nutrition, arterial congestion, venous
congestion, capillary congestion, astheny, &c., without being
acquainted with a single remedy by which they could reach
so visionary an object. It was ostentation that induced them
to attempt these cures which could not be advantageous to the
patients.

Every appearance of treating disease effectively and to the
purpose, disappears in their manner of *associating* various
medicinal substances to constitute what they call a *prescription*, and time has not only rendered this association sacred,
but *has converted it into a law*. They place at the head of this
recipe, under the name of basis, a medicine that is not at all
known in regard to the extent of its medicinal effects, but

---

* In the treatise "On the Sources of the Old Materia Medica," in the
third part of my Materia Medica.

which they think ought to subdue the principal character of
the disease admitted by the physician ; they add to this one or
two substances equally unknown in respect of their operation
on the system, and which they destine either to fulfil some accessory indication, or to increase the action of the basis ; they
then add a pretended corrective, of whose special medicinal
virtues they have no better knowledge ; they *mix* the whole
together, sometimes adding either a syrup, or a distilled water,
which likewise possess distinct medicinal properties, and imagine that each ingredient of the mixture will perform, in the
diseased body, the part that has been assigned to it by the
imagination, without allowing itself to be disturbed or led
astray by the other articles that accompany it:—a result which
no one could reasonably expect. One of these ingredients destroys, either partly or wholly, the operation of the other, or
gives to it, as well as to the remainder, a different mode of
action altogether which had never been thought of, so that the
effects calculated on, could *not possibly* take place. This inexplicable enigma of mixtures *often* produces that which
neither was nor could have been expected, a *new modification
of the disease,* which is not observed amidst the tumult of
symptoms, but which becomes permanent by the prolonged
use of the prescription. Consequently, a factitious malady,
joining itself to the original one, aggravates the primitive disease, or if the patient does not use the same prescription for
a long time, if one or several be crowded upon him successively, composed of different ingredients, *greater debility will at
least* ensue, because the substances which are prescribed in
such a case have generally little or no direct reference to the
principal malady, and only make a useless attack upon those
points against which its assaults have been the least directed.

Though the action of every medicine on the human body
should already have been discovered, still the physician who
writes the prescription does not often know the effect of one in
a hundred. Mixing several drugs together, some of which
are already compounds, and their separate effects imperfectly
known, in order that such a confused mixture should be swallowed by the patient in large and frequent doses, and then to
expect from it a certain curative effect, is an absurdity evident

to every unprejudiced* and reflecting individual. The result
is consequently the reverse of that which they expect to take
place in so precise a manner ; changes certainly take place,
but not one among them is either good or conformable to the
object that is to be attained.

* Even among the ordinary schools of medicine, there have been persons
who discovered the absurdity of mixing medicines, although they themselves
followed this eternal routine which their own reason condemned. Marcus
Herz expresses himself (Hufeland's Journal, II., p. 33) on this subject in
the following terms :—"When we wish to remove inflammation, we do not
employ either nitre, sal ammoniac, or vegetable acids, singly, but we usually
mix up several antiphlogistics, or use them altogether at the same time. If
we have to contend against putridity, we are not content with administering,
in large quantities, one of the known antiseptics, cinchona, mineral acids,
arnica, serpentaria, &c., to attain the object we have in view ; but we prefer
mixing up several of them together, having a greater reliance upon their combined action ; or, not knowing which of them would act most suitably in the
existing case, we accumulate a variety of incompatible substances, and abandon to chance the care of producing, by means of one or the other of them, the
relief we designed to afford. Thus, it is rare that, by the aid of a single
medicine, we excite perspiration, purify the blood, (?) dissolve obstructions,
provoke expectoration, or even effect purgation. To arrive at these results,
our prescriptions are always complicated; they are scarcely ever simple and
pure : *consequently they cannot be regarded as experiments relative to the
effects of the various substances that enter into their composition.* In fact,
we learnedly establish, among the medicines in our recipes, a hierarchy, and
we call that one the *basis* to which we (properly speaking) confide the effect,
giving to others the names of *adjuvants, corrigents,* &c. But it is evident
that mere arbitrary will has, for the most part, been the occasion of such a
classification. The adjuvants contribute, as well as the basis, to the entire
effect, although, in the absence of a scale of measurement, we cannot determine to what degree they may have participated. The influence of the corrigents over the virtues of the other medicines, likewise, cannot be wholly
indifferent; they must either increase or diminish them, or give them another
direction. The salutary change which we effect by the aid of such a prescription, ought then always to be considered as the result of its whole contents taken collectively, *and we can never come to any certain conclusion
upon the individual efficacy of any one of the ingredients of which it is composed. In short, we are but too slightly acquainted with that which is essential to be known of all medicines, and our knowledge with regard to the affini-
ties which they enter into, when mixed up together, is too limited for us to
be able to say, with any degree of certainty, what will be the mode or degree
of action of a subject even the most insignificant in appearance, when introduced into the human body, combined with other substances.*"

I should like very much to see that which is called *a cure*, by a man working thus blindly in the bodies of his fellow-creatures.

The restoration of health is to be expected only by cherishing the due activity of the vital principle yet remaining with the patient, by means of remedies suitable for that purpose, and not by debilitating the system, *secundum artem*, almost to the extinction of life. This is a method, however, not unfrequent with the old school on commencing the treatment of chronic diseases: they operate by means of medicines which harass the patient, expend the animal fluids, exhaust the strength, and shorten life! can they be said to save while they thus destroy? and can they be said to exercise any other than a hurtful art? They act, *lege artis*, as contrary to their professed aim as possible, and practise ἀλλᾶα, that is to say, the very reverse of what they ought to do. Can they deserve commendation? In modern times, indeed, this school have gone to great excesses in frustrating the end of all true medical treatment, as every impartial observer must acknowledge, and as physicians of their own (when their consciences are awakened, like that of Krueger Hansen) will confess, before the world.

———

Observation, reflection, and experience, have unfolded to me, that, in opposition to the old allœopathic method, the best and true method of cure is founded on the principle, *similia similibus curantur.* To cure in a mild, prompt, safe, and durable manner, it is necessary to choose in each case a medicine that will excite an affection similar (ὅμοιον πάθος) to that against which it is employed.

Until the present time, no person has ever inculcated this homœopathic mode of treatment, and yet more, no one has ever put it into practice. But if this is the only true method, (of which every one may be convinced with myself,) we ought to discover sensible traces of it in every epoch of the art, although its true character may have been unknown during thousands of years. And such has, in reality, been the case.*

In all ages, the diseases which have been cured by medicines, in a prompt, perfect, durable, and manifest manner, and which were not indebted for their cure to any accidental circumstance, or to the accomplishment of the natural revolution of the acute disease, or to the circumstance of the bodily powers having gradually regained a preponderance by means of an allœopathic or antipathic treatment, (for being cured directly differs greatly from being cured indirectly;) these diseases, I say, have yielded, although without the knowledge of the physician, to a homœopathic remedy, that is to say, to a remedy in itself capable of exciting a morbid state similar to that whose removal it effected.

Even in an effectual cure that had been performed by the aid of mixed medicines, (of which there are but few examples,) it has been discovered, that the medicine whose action dominated over that of the others was always of a homœopathic nature. But this fact presents itself to us still more evidently in certain cases, where physicians performed a speedy cure by the aid of a single remedy, in violation of the custom that admitted none other but mixed medicines in the form of a prescription. Here we see, to our astonishment, that the cure was always the effect of a single medicinal substance, capable of itself to produce an affection similar to that under which the patient laboured, although the physician did not know what he was doing, and only acted thus in forgetfulness of the precepts of his own school. He gave a medicine, where, according to the established laws of therapeutics, he should have administered exactly a contrary one, and by these means alone his patients were promptly cured.

---

* For Truth, like the infinitely wise and gracious God, is eternal. Men may disregard it for a time, until the period arrives when its rays, according to the determination of Heaven, shall irresistibly break through the mists of prejudice, and, like Aurora and the opening day, shed a beneficent light, clear and inextinguishable, over the generations of men.

I shall here relate some examples of these homœopathic cures, which find a clear and precise interpretation in the homœopathic doctrine now discovered and acknowledged, but which we are by no means to regard as arguments in favour of the latter, because it stands firm without the aid of any such support.*

The author of the treatise on epidemic diseases, (ἐπιδημιῶν) (attributed to Hippocrates,) at the commencement of lib. 5. mentions a case of *cholera morbus* that resisted every remedy, and which he cured by means of veratrum album alone, which, however, excites *cholera* of itself, as witnessed by Forestus, Ledelius, Reimann, and many others.†

The English *sweating sickness*, which first exhibited itself in the year 1485, and which, more murderous than the plague itself, carried off in the commencement, (as testified by Willis,) ninety-nine patients out of a hundred, could not be subdued until such time as they had learned to administer *sudorifics* to patients. Since that time, as Sennertus‡ observes, few persons died of it.

A case of *dysentery*, which lasted several years, threatening the patient with inevitable death, and against which every other medicine had been tried without success, was, to the

---

* If, in the cases which will be cited here, the doses of medicine exceeded those which the safe homœopathic doctrine prescribes, they were, of course, very naturally attended with the same degree of danger which usually results from all homœopathic agents when administered in large doses. However, it often happens, from various causes, which cannot at all times be discovered, that even very large doses of homœopathic medicines effect a cure, without causing any notable injury; either from the vegetable substance having lost a part of its strength, or because abundant evacuations ensued, which destroyed the greater part of the effects of the remedy; or, finally, because the stomach had received at the same time other substances, which, acting as an antidote, lessened the strength of the dose.

† P. FORESTUS, xviii. *obs.* 44.—LEDELIUS, *Misc. Nat. Cur. dec.* iii. *ann. i. obs.* 65.—REIMANN, *Bresl. Samml.* 1724, 535. In this, and in all the examples that follow, I have purposely abstained from reporting either my own observations or those of my adherents upon the special effects of each individual medicine, but merely those of the physicians of times past. My object for acting in this manner is, to show that the art of curing homœopathically might have been discovered before my time.

‡ De Febribus, iv. cap. 15.

great surprise of Fischer,* (but not to mine,) cured in a speedy and permanent manner by a *purgative* administered by an empiric.

Murray, (whom I selected from numerous other authorities,) together with daily experience, informs us, that among the symptoms produced by the use of *tobacco*, those of *vertigo, nausea,* and *anxiety,* are the principal. Whereas Diemerbroeck,† when attacked with those very symptoms of vertigo, nausea, and anxiety, in the course of his close attendance on the victims of epidemic diseases in Holland, removed them by the use of the pipe.

The hurtful effects which some writers (among others Georgi‡) ascribe to the use of the *agaricus muscarius*, by the inhabitants of Kamtschatka, and which consist of *tremors, convulsions,* and *epilepsy,* became a salutary remedy in the hands of C. G. Whistling,§ who used this mushroom with success in cases of convulsions accompanied with tremor ; likewise in those of J. C. Bernhardt,‖ who used it with success in a species of epilepsy.

The remark made by Murray,** that oil of *aniseed* allays pains of the stomach and flatulent colic caused by purgatives, ought not to surprise us, knowing that J. P. Albrecht†† has observed *pains in the stomach* produced by this liquid ; and P. Forestus‡‡ *violent colic* likewise caused by its administration.

If F. Hoffman praises the efficacy of *millefoil* in various cases of *hemorrhage ;* if G. E. Stahl, Buchwalk and Löseke have found this plan useful in excessive hemorrhoidal flux ; if Quarin and the editors of the *Bresslauer Sammlungen* speak of the cure it has effected of hemoptysis ; and finally, if Thomasius (according to Haller) has used it successfully in uterine

---

* In Hufeland's Journal für Practische, Arzneikunde, vol. x. iv. p. 127.

† Tract de Peste, Amsterdam, 1665, p. 273.

‡ Beschreibung aller Nationen des Russischen Reiĉhs, (A Description of all the Nations of the Russian Empire,) pp. 78, 267, 281, 321, 329, 352.

§ Diss. de Virt. Agaric. Musc. Jena, 1718, p. 13.

‖ Chym. Vers. und Erfahrungen, Leipzig, 1754, obs. 5, p. 324. GRUNER, De Viribus Agar. Musc. Jena, 1778, p. 13.

** Appar. Medic., 2d edit. I, p. 429, 430.

†† Misc. Nat. Cur. dec. ii. ann. 8, obs. 169.

‡‡ Observat. et. Curationes, lib 21.

hemorrhage ; these cures are evidently owing to the power possessed by the plant, of exciting of itself *hemorrhage* and *hematuria,* as observed by G. Hoffman,* and more especially of producing *epistaxis* as confirmed by Boecler.†

Scovolo,‡ among many others, cured a case where the urinary discharge was purulent, by *arbutus uva ursi ;* which never could have been performed if this plant had not the property of exciting *heat in the urinary passage with discharge of a mucous urine,* as seen by Sauvages.§

And though the frequent experience of Stoerck, Marges, Planchon, Du Monceau, F. C. Junker, Schinz, Ehrmann, and others, had not already established the fact, that *colchicum autumnale* cures a species of dropsy, still this faculty was to have been expected from it, by reason of the particular power which it possesses of *diminishing the urinary secretion,* and *of exciting at the same time a continual desire to pass water.* It likewise causes the flow of a *small quantity of urine, of a fiery red colour,* as witnessed by Stoerck‖ and de Berge.** The cure of an asthma attended with hypochondriasis effected by Göritz†† by means of colchicum, and that of an asthma complicated with an apparent hydrothorax, performed by Stoerck‡‡ with the same substance, were evidently grounded upon the homœopathic property which it possesses, of exciting by itself *asthma* and *dyspnœa,* as witnessed by de Berge.§§

Muralto‖‖ has seen what we may witness every day, viz., that *jalap,* besides creating *gripes of the stomach,* also causes *great uneasiness* and *agitation.* Every physician acquainted with the facts upon which homœopathy rests, will find it perfectly natural, that the power so justly ascribed to this medi-

* De Medicam. Officin.   Leyden, 1738.
† Cynosura Mat. Med. Cont., p. 552.
‡ In Girardi, de uva ursi.   Padua, 1764.
§ Nosolog., iii. p. 200.
‖ Libellus de Colchico.   Vienna, 1763, p. 12.
** Journal de Médecine, xxii.
†† A. E. Büchner, Miscell. Phys. Med. Mathem. Ann. 1728, Jul. pp. 1212, 1213.   Erfurt, 1732.
‡‡ Ibid. cas. 11, 13.   Cont. cas. 4, 9.
§§ Ibid. loc. cit.
‖‖ Misc. Nat. Cur. dec. ii. a. 7, obs. 112.

cine by G. W. Wedel,* of allaying the gripes, restlessness, and screaming which are so frequent in young children, and of restoring them to tranquil repose, arises from homœopathic influence.

It is also known and has been attested by Murray, Hillary, and Spielmann, that *senna* occasions a kind of colic, and produces, according to C. Hoffman† and F. Hoffman,‡ *flatulency* and *agitation of the blood*,§ ordinary causes of *insomnolency*. It was this innate homœopathic virtue of senna, which enabled Detharding‖ to cure with its aid patients afflicted with violent colic and insomnolency.

Stoerck, who had so intimate a knowledge of medicines, was on the point of discovering that the bad effects of the *dictamnus*, which, as he observed himself, sometimes provokes a *mucous discharge from the vagina*,** arose from the very same properties in this root by virtue of which he cured a leucorrhœa of long standing.††

Stoerck, in like manner, should not have been astonished when curing a general chronic eruption, (humid, phagedenic and psoric,) with the *clematis*,‡‡ having himself ascertained §§ that this plant has the power of producing a *psoric eruption over the whole body*.

If, according to Murray,‖‖ the *euphrasia* cures lippitudo and a certain form of ophthalmy, how could it otherwise have produced this effect, but by the faculty it possesses of exciting a kind *of inflammation in the eyes*, as has been remarked by Lobelius ?***

According to J. H. Lange,††† the *nutmeg* has been found

---

* Opiolog. lib. 1, p. 1, cap. ii. p. 38
† De Medicin. Officin. lib. 1. cap. 36.
‡ Diss. de Manna, § 16.
§ Murray, loc. cit. ii. p. 507, 2d edit.
‖ Ephem. Nat. Cur. cent. 10, obs. 76.
** Lib. de Flamm. Jovis. Vienna, 1769, cap. 2.
†† Ibid.
‡‡ Lib. de Flamm. Jovis. Vienna, 1769, cap. 13.
§§ Ibid. p. 33.
‖‖ Appar. Medic. 11, p. 221, 2d edit.
*** Stirp. Adversar. p. 219.
††† Domest. Brunsvic. p. 136.

efficacious in hysterical fainting fits. The sole natural cause
of this phenomenon is homœopathic, and can be attributed to
no other circumstance but that the nutmeg, when given in
strong doses to a man in health, produces, according to J.
Schmid* and Cullen,† *suspension of the senses and general insensibility.*

The old practice of applying *rose-water* externally in oph-
thalmic diseases, looks like a tacit avowal, that there exists in
the leaves of the rose some curative power for diseases of the
eye. This is founded upon the homœopathic virtue which the
rose possesses, of exciting by itself a species of *ophthalmia* in
persons who are in health, an effect which Echtius,‡ Ledelius,§ and Rau,‖ actually saw it produce.

If, according to Pet. Rossi,** Van Mons,†† J. Monti,‡‡
Sybel,§§ and others, the *Rhus toxicodendron* and *radicans* have
the faculty of producing *pimples which gradually cover the entire body,* it may be easily peceived how it could effect an
homœopathic cure of various kinds of herpes, which it really
has done, according to information furnished by Dufresnoy and
Van Mons. What could have bestowed upon this plant (as in
a case cited by Alderson‖‖) the power of curing a paralysis of
the lower extremities, attended with weakness of the intellectual organs, if it did not of itself evidently possess the
faculty of *depressing the muscular powers* by acting on the
imagination of the patient to such a degree as to make him
believe that he is at the point of death, as in a case witnessed
by Zadig.***

The *dulcamara,* according to Carrère,††† has cured the most

---

* Misc. Nat. Cur. dec. ii. ann. 2, obs. 20.
† Arzneimittellehre, ii. p. 233.
‡ In Adami, Vita Medic. p. 72.
§ Misc. Nat. Curios. dec. ii. ann. 2, obs. 140.
‖ Rau, über den Werth des Homœop. Heilverfahrens, p. 73.
** Observ. de Nonnullis Plantis, quæ pro venenatis habentur. Pisis, 1767.
†† In Dufresnoy Ueber den wurzelnden Sumach, p. 206.
‡‡ Acta Instit. Bonon. sc. et art. iii. p. 165.
§§ In Med. Annalen, 1811, July.
‖‖ In Samml. aus. Abh. f. pr. Aerzte, xviii. 1.
*** In Hufeland's Journal der Prakt. Arzneik. v. p. 3.
††† Carrère (and Starcke,) Abhandl. ueber die Eigenschaften des Nacht-

violent diseases emanating from colds, which could result from
no other cause but that this herb, in cold and damp weather,
frequently produces *similar affections to those which arise from
colds*, as Carrère himself has observed,* and likewise Starcke.†
—Fritze‡ saw the dulcamara produce *convulsions*, and De
Haen§ witnessed the *very same effects, attended with delirium ;*
on the other hand, convulsions attended with delirium have
yielded to small doses of the dulcamara, administered by the
latter physician.‖—It were vain to seek amid the vast empire
of hypotheses the cause that renders the dulcamara so efficacious in a species of herpes, as witnessed by Carrère,** Fouquet,†† and Poupart.‡‡ Nature, which requires the aid of
homœopathy to perform a safe cure, sufficiently explains the
cause, in the faculty possessed by the dulcamara of producing
a certain species of herpes. Carrère saw the use of this plant
excite herpetic eruptions which covered the entire body during a fortnight ;§§ and on another occasion where it produced
the same *on the hands ;*‖‖ and a third time where it fixed itself
on the *labia pudendi.***

Rucker††† saw the *solanum nigrum* produce *swelling of the
entire body.* This is the reason that Gatacker‡‡‡ and Cirillo§§§
succeeded in curing with its aid (homœopathically) a species
of dropsy.

schattens oder Bittersuesses. Jena, 1786, pp. 20–23. (Treatise on the
Properties of the Woody Nightshade or Bitter-sweet.)
* Ibid.
† In Carrère, Ibid. p. 140, 249.
‡ Annalen des Klinischen Instituts, iii. p. 45.
§ Ratio Medendi. Tom. iv. p. 228.
‖ Ibid.,where he says : " Dulco-amaræ stipites majori dosi convulsiones et
deliria excitant, moderata vero spasmos, convulsionesque solvunt." How
near was De Haen to the discovery of the law of healing the most conform-
able to nature !
** Ratio Medendi. Tom. iv. p.92.
†† In Razouz, Tables Nosologiques, p. 275.
‡‡ Traité des Dartres. Paris, 1782, pp. 184, 192.
§§ Ibid. p. 96.   ‖‖ Ibid. p. 149.   *** Ibid. p. 164.
††† Commerc. Liter. Noric. 1731, p. 372.
‡‡‡ Versuche & Bemerk. der Edinb. Gesellschaft, Altenburg, 1762, vii.
pp. 95, 98.
§§§ Consult. Medichi. Tom. iii. Naples, 1738, 4to.

Boerhaave,[*] Sydenham,[†] and Radcliffe,[‡] cured another species of dropsy with the aid of the *sambucus niger*, because, as Haller[§] informs us, this plant causes an *œdematous swelling* when applied externally.

De Haen,[‖] Sarcone,[**] and Pringle[††] have rendered due homage to truth and experience, by declaring freely, that they cured pleurisy with the *scilla maritima*, a root which, on account of its excessive acrid properties, ought to be forbidden in a disease of this nature, where, according to the received method, only sedative, relaxing, and refrigerant remedies are admissible. The disease in question subsided, nevertheless, under the influence of the squill, on homœopathic principles; for T. C. Wagner[‡‡] formerly saw the action of this plant alone produce *pleurisy* and *inflammation of the lungs*.

A great many practitioners, D. Crueger, Ray, Kellner, Kaaw Boerhaave, and others,[§§] have observed that the *daturà stramonium* excites a singular kind of delirium and *convulsions*. It is precisely this faculty that enabled physicians to cure with its aid, demonomania[‖‖] (fantastic madness, attended with spasms of the limbs) and other convulsions, as performed by Sidren[***] and Wedenberg.[†††] If in the hands of Sidren[‡‡‡] it cured two cases of chorea, one of which had been occasioned by fright, and the other by mercurial vapour, it was because it possessed the faculty of exciting involuntary movements of the limbs, as observed by Kaaw Boerhaave, and Lobstein. Numerous observations, and among others those made by Schenk, have shown us that it can destroy consciousness and

---

* Historia Plantarum, P. I. p. 207. † Opera, p. 496.
‡ In Haller, Arzneimittellehre, p. 349.
§ In Vicat, Plantes vénéneuses, p. 125.
‖ Ratio Medendi, P. I. p. 13.
** History of Diseases in Naples, vol. i. § 175.
†† Obs. on the Diseases of the Army, ed. 7, § 143.
‡‡ Observationes Clinicæ. Lubec, 1737.
§§ C. Crueger, in Misc. Nat. Cur., dec. iii. ann. 2, obs. 88.—Boerhaave, Impetum Faciens.—Leiden, 1745, p. 282.—Kellner, in the Bresl. Samml. 172.
‖‖ Veckoskrift for Laekare, iv. p. 40, et seq.
*** Diss. de Stramonii Usu in Malis Convulsivis. Upsal, 1793.
††† Ibid.
‡‡‡ Diss. Morborum Casus, spec. i. Upsal, 1785.

recollection in a very short time; therefore, it ought not to surprise us, if, according to the testimony of Sauvages and Schinz, it possesses the faculty of curing a weak memory. By the same rule, Schmalz* succeeded in curing with the aid of this plant a case of melancholy, alternating with madness, because, according to a Costa,† it has the power of exciting such alternate mental aberrations when administered to a person in health.

Percival, Stahl, Quarin,‡ and many other physicians, have observed that *cinchona* occasions *oppression of the stomach*. Others, (Morton, Friborg, Bauer, and Quarin,) have seen this substance produce *vomiting* and *diarrhœa*, (D. Crueger and Morton) *syncope*; some an excessive *debility*, many (Thomson, Richard, Stahl, and C. E. Fisher) a kind of *jaundice*; (Quarin and Fischer) *bitterness of the mouth*; and yet others, *tension of the belly*. And it is precisely when these complicated evils occur in intermittent fevers, that Torti and Cleghorn recommend the use of cinchona alone. The advantageous effects of this bark in cases of exhaustion, indigestion, and loss of appetite resulting from acute fevers, (particularly when the latter have been treated by venesection, evacuants and debilitants,) are founded upon the faculty which it possesses of *depressing excessively the vital powers, producing mental and bodily exhaustion, indigestion, and loss of appetite*, as observed by Cleghorn, Friborg, Crueger, Romberg, Stahl, Thomson, and others.§

How would it have been possible to stop hemorrhages with *ipecacuanha*, as effected by Baglivi, Barbeyrac, Gianella, Dalberg, Bergius, and others, if this medicine did not of itself possess the faculty of exciting hemorrhage homœopathically?— as Murray, Scott, and Geoffroy‖ have witnessed. How could it be so efficacious in asthma, and particularly in spasmodic asthma, as it is described to have been, by Akenside,** Meyer,††

---

* Chir. und Medic. Vorfälle. Leipzig, 1784, p. 178.

† In P. Schenck, lib. 1, obs. 139.

‡ Quoted in my Mat. Med. iii.

§ Mat. Med. iii.   ‖ Ibid. pp. 184, 185.

** Medic. Transact. I. No. 7, p. 39.

†† Diss. de Ipecac. refracta dosi usu, p. 34.

Bang,* Stoll,† Fouquet,‡ and Ranoë,§ if it did not of itself produce (without exciting any evacuation) *asthma*, and *spasmodic asthma* in particular, as Murray,‖ Geoffroy,** and Scott†† have seen it call forth? Can any clearer hints be required, that medicines ought to be applied to the cure of diseases according to the morbid effects which they produce?

It would be impossible to conceive why the *Faba Ignatia* could be so efficacious in a kind of convulsions, as we are assured it is, by Hermann,‡‡ Valentin,§§ and an anonymous writer,‖‖ if it did not possess the power of exciting similar *convulsions*, as witnessed by Bergius,*** Camelli,††† and Durius.‡‡‡

Persons who have received a *blow* or a *contusion*, feel pains in the side, a desire to vomit, spasmodic, lancinating and burning pain in the hypochondres, all of which are accompanied with anxiety, tremors, and involuntary starts, similar to those produced by an electric shock, formication in the parts that have received the injury, &c. As the *arnica montana* produces similar symptoms, according to the observations of Meza, Vicat, Crichton, Collins, Aaskow, Stoll, and J. C. Lange;§§§ it may be easily conceived on what account this plant cures the effects of a blow, fall, or contusion, and consequently the malady itself occasioned by such a contusion, as experienced by a host of physicians, and even whole nations, for centuries past.

Among the effects which *belladonna* excites when administered to a person in sound health, are symptoms which, taken collectively, present an image greatly resembling that species

* Praxis Medica, p. 346.
† Prælectiones, p. 221.
‡ Journal de Médecine, tom. 62, p. 137.
§ In Act. Reg. Soc. Med. Hafn., ii. p. 163, iii. p. 361.
‖ Medic. Pract. Bibl., p. 237.
** Traité de la Matière Médicale, ii. p. 157.
†† In Med. Comment. of Edinb. iv. p. 74.
‡‡ Cynosura Mat. Med. ii. p. 231.
§§ Hist. Simplic. Reform. p. 194, § 4.
‖‖ In Act. Berol. dec. ii. vol. x. p. 12.
*** Materia Medica, p. 150.
††† Philos. Trans. vol. xxi. No. 250.
‡‡‡ Miscell. Nat. Cur. dec. iii. ann. 9, 10.
§§§ See my Mat. Medica, i.

of *hydrophobia* and *rabies canina* which Mayerne,[*] Münch,[†] Buchholz,[‡] and Neimike,[§] cured in a perfect manner with this plant homœopathically.[||] *The patient in vain endeavours to sleep, the respiration is embarrassed, he is consumed by a burning thirst, attended with anxiety; the moment any liquids are presented to him, he rejects them with violence; his countenance becomes red, his eyes fixed and sparkling,* (as observed by F. C. Grimm;) *he experiences a feeling of suffocation while drinking,* with excessive thirst, (according to E. Camerarius and Sauter;) for the most part he is *incapable of swallowing anything,* (as affirmed by May, Lottinger, Sicelius, Buchave, D'Hermont, Manetti, Vicat, and Cullen;) he is *alternately actuated by terror and a desire to bite the persons who are near him,* (as seen by Sauter, Dumoulin, Buchave, and Mardorf;) *he spits everywhere around him,* (according to Sauter;) *he endeavours to make his escape,* (as we are informed by Dumoulin, E. Gmelin, and Buc'hoz;) and a continual agility of the body is predominant, (as witnessed by Boucher E. Gmelin, and Sauter.)[**]   Belladonna has also effected the cure of different kinds of madness and melancholy, as in the cases reported by Evers, Schmucker, Schmalz, the two Münches, and many others, because it possesses the faculty of producing different kinds of *insanity* like those mental diseases caused by belladonna, which are noted by Rau, Grimm, Hasenest, Mardorf, Hoyer, Dillenius, and

[*] Praxeos in Morbis internis Syntagma alterum. Augustæ Vindelicorum, 1697, p. 136.

[†] Beobachtungen bei angewendeter Belladonne bei den Menschen. Stendal, 1789.

[‡] Heilsame Wirkungen der Belladonne in ausgebrochener Wuth. Erfurt, 1785.

[§] In J. H. Münch's Beobachtungen, Th. i. p. 74.

[||] If belladonna has frequently failed in cases of decided rabies, we ought to remember that it cannot cure in such instances, but by its faculty of producing effects similar to those of the malady itself, and that, consequently, it ought not to be administered but in the smallest possible doses, as will be shown in the Organon, (§ 275–283.) In general, it has been administered in very large doses, so that the patients *necessarily* died, not of the disease, but of the remedy. However, there may exist more than one degree or species of hydrophobia and rabies, and consequently (according to the diversity of the symptoms) the most suitable homœopathic remedy may be sometimes hyosciamus, and sometimes stramonium.

[**] The places from these authors are referred to in my Mat. Medica, i.

others.* Henning,† after vainly endeavouring, during three months, to cure a case of amaurosis with coloured spots before the eyes, by a variety of medicines, was at length struck with the idea that this malady might perhaps be occasioned by gout, although the patient had never experienced the slightest attack ; and upon this supposition he was by chance induced to prescribe belladonna,‡ which effected a speedy cure free from any inconvenience. He would undoubtedly have made choice of this remedy at the commencement, had he known that it was not possible to perform a cure but by the aid of a remedy which produces symptoms similar to those of the disease itself ; and that, according to the infallible law of nature, belladonna could not fail to cure this case homœopathically, since, by the testimony of Sauter§ and Buchholz,‖ it excites, of itself, a species of *amaurosis with coloured spots before the eyes.*

The *hyosciamus* has cured spasms which strongly resembled epilepsy ; as witnessed by Mayerne,** Stoerck, Collin, and others. It produces this effect by the very same power that it excites *convulsions similar to those of epilepsy,* as observed in the writings of E. Camerarius, C. Seliger, Hünerwolf, A. Hamilton, Planchon, Acosta, and others.††

Fothergill,‡‡ Stoerck, Hellwig, and Ofterdinger, have used hyosciamus with success in certain kinds of mental derangement. But the use of it would have been attended with equal success in the hands of many other physicians, had they confined it to the cure of that species of mental alienation which hyosciamus is capable of producing in its primitive effects, viz., a kind of derangement with stupefaction, that Van Helmont, Medel, J. G. Gmelin, La Serre, Hünerwolf, A. Hamilton, Kiernander, J. Stedmann, Tozzetti, J. Faber, and Wendt saw produced by the action of this plant.§§

* Referred to in my Materia Medica, i.
† In-Hufeland's Journal, xxv. iv. pp. 70, 74.
‡ Mere conjecture alone has led physicians to rank belladonna among the remedies for gout. The disease which could, with justice, arrogate to itself the name of gout, never will nor can be cured by belladonna.
§ In Hufeland's Journal, xi.
‖ Ibid. vol. i. p. 252.   ** Prax. Med. p. 28.
†† See my Materia Medica, vol. iv.
‡‡ Memoirs of Med. Soc. of London, i. pp. 310, 314.
§§ See my Materia Medica, vol. iv.

By taking the effects of hyosciamus collectively which the latter observers have seen it produce, they present a picture of hysteria arrived at a considerable height. We also find in J. A. P. Gessner, Stoerck, and in the Act. Nat. Cur.,* that a case of hysteria, which bore great resemblance to the above mentioned, was cured by the use of this plant.

Schenkbecher† would never have succeeded in curing a vertigo of twenty years' standing, if this plant did not possess, in a very high degree, the power of creating generally an analogous state, as attested by Hünerwolf, Blom, Navier, Planchon, Sloane, Stedmann, Greding, Wepfer, Vicat, and Bernigau.‡

A man, who became deranged through jealousy, was for a long time tormented by Mayer Abramson§ with remedies that produced no effect on him, when, under the name of a soporific, he one day administered *hyosciamus*, which cured him speedily. Had he known that this plant excites *jealousy* and *madness* in persons who are in health,‖ and had he been acquainted with the homœopathic law, (the sole natural basis of therapeutics,) he would have been able to administer hyosciamus from the very commencement with perfect confidence, and thus have avoided fatiguing the patient with remedies which (not being homœopathic) could be of no manner of service to him.

The mixed prescriptions which were employed for a long time with the greatest success by Hecker** in a case of *spasmodic constriction of the eyelids*, would have proved ineffectual, if some happy chance had not included hyosciamus, which, according to Wepfer,†† excites a similar affection in persons who are in sound health.

Neither did Withering‡ succeed in curing a spasmodic constriction of the pharynx, with inability to swallow, until he

* IV. obs. 8.
† Von der Kinkina, Schierling, Bilsenkraut, &c. Riga, 1769, p. 162.
‡ See my Mat. Medica, vol. iv.
§ In Hufeland's Journal, xix. ii. p. 60.
‖ See my Mat. Medica, vol. iv.
** Hufeland's Journal, d. pr. Arzneik. i. p. 354.
†† De Cicuta Aquatica. Basil. 1716, p. 320.
‡‡ Edinb. Med. Comment. Dec. ii. B. vi. p. 263.

administered hyosciamus, whose special action consists of causing a *spasmodic constriction of the throat, with the impossibility of swallowing,* an effect which Tozzetti, Hamilton, Bernigau, Sauvages, and Hünerwolf* have seen it produce in a very high degree.

How could *camphor* produce such salutary effects as the veracious Huxham† says it does, in the so-called slow nervous fevers, where the temperature of the body is decreased, where the sensibility is depressed, and the vital powers greatly diminished, if the result of its immediate action upon the body did not produce a *state similar in every respect* to the latter, as observed by G. Alexander, Cullen, and F. Hoffman?‡

Spirituous *wines*, administered in small doses, have cured, homœopathically, *fevers* that were purely *inflammatory.* C. Crivellati,§ H. Augenius,‖ A. Mundella,** and two anonymous writers,†† have afforded us the proofs. Asclepiades‡‡ on one occasion cured an *inflammation of the brain* by administering a *small quantity of wine.* A case of feverish delirium like an insensible drunkenness, attended with stertorous breathing, similar to that state of deep intoxication which wine produces, was cured in a single night by *wine* which Rademacher§§ administered to the patient. Can any one deny the power of a medicinal irritation analogous to the disease itself (*similia similibus*) in either of these cases?

A strong infusion of *tea* produces *anxiety* and *palpitation of the heart* in persons who are not in the habit of drinking it; on the other hand, if taken in small doses, it is an excellent remedy against such symptoms when produced by other causes, as testified by G. L. Rau.‖‖

---

* See my Materia Medica, vol. iv. pp. 38, 39.
† Opera, t. i. p. 172 ; t. ii. p. 84.
‡ See my Materia Medica, vol. iv.
§ Trattato dell' uso e modo di dare il vino nelle febri acute. Rome, 1600.
‖ Epist. t. ii. lib. ii. ep. 8.
** Epist. 14. Basil, 1538.
†† Eph. Nat. Cur. dec. ii. ann. 2, obs. 53. Gazette de Santé, 1788.
‡‡ Cœl. Aurelianus, Acut. lib. i. c. 16.
§§ In Hufeland's Journal, xvi. i. p. 92.
‖‖ Ueber den Werth des Homœopathischen Heilverfahrens. Heidelberg, 1824, p. 75.

A case resembling the agonies of death, in which the patient was convulsed to such a degree as to deprive him of his senses, alternating with attacks of spasmodic breathing, sometimes also sobbing and stertorous respiration, with icy coldness of the face and body, lividity of the feet and hands, and feebleness of the pulse, (a state perfectly analogous to the whole of the symptoms which Schweikert and others saw produced by the use of *opium*,)* was at first treated unsuccessfully by Stütz† with ammonia, but afterwards cured in a speedy and permanent manner with *opium*. In this instance, could any one fail to discover the homœopathic method brought into action without the knowledge of the person who employed it? According to Vicat, J. C. Grimm, and others,‡ opium also produces *a powerful and almost irresistible tendency to sleep, accompanied by profuse perspiration and delirium.* This was the reason why Osthoff§ was afraid to administer it in cases of epidemic fever which exhibited *similar symptoms,* for the principles of the system which he pursued prohibited the use of it under such circumstances. (The poor system!) However, after having exhausted in vain all the known remedies, and seeing his patients at the point of death, he resolved, at all hazards, to administer a small quantity of opium, whose effects proved salutary, as they always must, according to the unerring law of homœopathy.

J. Lind‖ likewise avows that "opium removes the complaints in the head, while the perspiration tediously breaks forth during the heat of the body; it relieves the head, destroys the burning febrile heat of the skin, softens it, and bathes its surface in a profuse perspiration. But Lind was not aware that this salutary effect of opium (contrary to the axioms of the school of medicine) is owing to the circumstance of its producing analogous morbid symptoms, when administered to a person in health. There has, nevertheless, here

* See my Materia Medica, vol. i.

† In Hufeland's Journal, x. iv.

‡ See my Materia Medica, vol. i.

§ In the Salzburg Med. Chirurg. Journal, 1805, iii. p. 110.

‖ Versuch über die Krankheiten denen die Europäer in heissen Klimaten unterworfen sind. Riga and Leipzig, 1773. (Treatise on the Diseases to which Europeans are subject in Warm Climates.)

and there been a physician, across whose mind this truth has passed like a flash of lightning, without ever giving birth to a suspicion of the laws of homœopathy. For example, Alston* says that *opium* is a remedy that excites heat, notwithstanding which, it certainly diminishes heat where it already exists. De la Guérène† administered opium in a case of fever attended with violent headache, tension and hardness of the pulse, dryness and roughness of the skin, burning heat, and hence difficult and debilitating perspirations, the exhalation of which was constantly interrupted by the extreme agitation of the patient; and was successful with it, because opium possesses the faculty of creating a feverish state in healthy persons, which is perfectly analogous, as asserted by many observers,‡ and of which he was ignorant. In a fever attended with coma, where the patient, deprived of speech, lay extended, the eyes open, the limbs stiff, the pulse small and intermittent, the respiration disturbed and stertorous, (all of which are symptoms perfectly similar to those which opium excites, according to the report of Delacroix, Rademacher, Crumpe, Pyl, Vicat, Sauvages and many others,§) this was the only substance which C. L. Hoffman‖ saw produce any good effects, *which were naturally a homœopathic result.* Wirthenson,** Sydenham,†† and Marcus,‡‡ have even succeeded in curing lethargic fevers with opium. A case of lethargy of which De Meza§§ effected a cure, would yield only to this substance, which, in such cases, acts homœopathically, since it produces lethargy of itself.

C. C. Matthäi,‖‖ in an obstinate case of nervous disease, where the principal symptoms were insensibility, and numbness of the arms, legs, and belly, after having for a long time

* In Edinb. Versuchen, v. p. 1, art. 12.
† In Römer's Annalen der Arzneimittellehre, I. ii. p. 6.
‡ See my Materia Medica, vol. i.
§ Ibid.
‖ Von Scharbock, Lustseuche, &c. Münster, 1787, p. 295.
** Opii vires fibras cordis debilitare, &c. Münster, 1775.
†† Opera, p. 654.
‡‡ Magazin für Thèrapie, I. i. p. 7.
§§ Act. Reg. Soc. Med. Hafn. iii. p. 202.
‖‖ In Struve's Triumph der Heilk. iii.

treated it with inappropriate, that is to say, non-homœopathic remedies, at length effected a cure by opium, which, according to Stütz, J. Young, and others,[*] excites similar symptoms of a very intense nature, and which, as every one must perceive, only succeeded on this occasion by homœopathic means. The cure of a case of lethargy which had already existed several days, and which Hufeland performed by the use of opium,[†] by what other law could this have been effected, if not by that of homœopathy, which has remained disregarded till the present time? In that peculiar species of epilepsy which never manifests itself but during sleep, De Haen discovered that it was not at all a sleep, but a lethargic stupor, with stertorous respiration, perfectly similar to that which opium produces in persons who are in health: it was by the means of opium alone that he transformed it into a natural and healthy sleep, while at the same time he delivered the patient of his epilepsy.[‡]

How would it be possible that opium, which of all vegetable substances is the one whose administration, in small doses, produces the most powerful and obstinate constipation, as a primary effect, should notwithstanding be a remedy the most to be relied upon in cases of constipation which endanger life, if it was not in virtue of the homœopathic law, so little known—that is to say, if nature had not decreed that medicines should subdue natural diseases by a special action on their part, which consists in producing an analogous affection? Opium, whose first effects are so powerful in constipating the bowels, was discovered by Tralles[§] to be the only cure in a case of ileus, which he had till then treated ineffectually with evacuants and other unappropriate remedies. Lentilius[‖] and G. W. Wedel,[**] Wirthenson, Bell, Heister, and Richter,[††] have

[*] See my Materia Medica, vol. i.
[†] In Hufeland's Journal, xii. i.
[‡] Ratio Medendi, V. p. 126.
[§] Opii usus et abusus, sect. ii. p. 260.
[‖] Eph. Nat. Cur. dec. iii. ann. i. app. p. 131.
[**] Opiologia, p. 120.
[††] Anfangsgründe der Wundarzneikunde, V. § 328.—Chronische Krankheiten. Berlin, 1816, ii. p. 220. (Rudiments of Surgery, V. § 328.—Chronic Diseases, Berlin, 1816, ii. p. 220.)

likewise confirmed the efficacy of opium, even when administered alone in this disease. The candid Bohn* was likewise convinced by experience that *nothing* but *opiates* would act as purgatives in the colic called *miserere;* and the celebrated Fr. Hoffman,† in the most dangerous cases of this nature, placed his sole reliance on opium, combined with the anodyne liquor called after his name. All the theories contained in the two hundred thousand volumes that have been written on medicine, would they be able to furnish us with a rational explanation of this and so many other similar facts, being ignorant of the therapeutic law of homœopathia? Have their doctrines conducted us to the discovery of this law of nature so clearly manifested in *every* perfect, speedy, and permanent cure—that is to say, have they taught us that when we use medicines in the treatment of diseases, it is necessary to take for a guide the resemblance of their effects upon a person in health, to the symptoms of those very diseases?

Rave‡ and Wedekind § have suppressed uterine hemorrhage with the aid of *sabina,* which, as every one knows, causes *uterine hemorrhage,* and consequently abortion with women who are in health. Could any one, in this case, fail to perceive the homœopathic law which ordains that we should cure *similia similibus?*

In that species of spasmodic asthma designated by the name of Millar, how could *musk* act almost specifically, if it did not of itself produce paroxysms of a spasmodic constriction of the chest without cough, as observed by F. Hoffman?‖

Could vaccination protect us from the small pox otherwise than homœopathically? Without mentioning any other traits of close resemblance which often exist between these two maladies, they have this in common—they generally appear but once during the course of a person's life; they leave behind cicatrices equally deep; they both occasion tumefaction of the axillary glands; a fever that is analogous; an inflamed areola around each pock; and finally, ophthalmia and convulsions.

* De Officio Medici.
† Medicin. rat. system. T. IV. p. ii. p. 297.
‡ Beobachtungen und Schlüsse, (Observations and Conclusions,) ii. p. 7.
§ In Hufeland's Journal, X. i. p. 77; and in his "Aufsaetzen," p. 278.
‖ Med. ration. system. iii. p. 92.

The cow-pock would even destroy the small-pox on its first appearance, that is to say, it would cure this already existing malady, if the intensity of the small-pox did not predominate over it. To produce this effect, then, it only wants that excess of power which, according to the law of nature, ought to *correspond* with the homœopathic resemblance, in order to effect a cure (§. 158). Vaccination, considered as a homœopathic remedy, cannot, therefore, prove efficacious except when employed previous to the appearance of the small-pox, which is the stronger of the two.

In this manner it excites a disease very analogous (and consequently homœopathic) to the small-pox, after whose course the human body, which, according to custom, can only be attacked once with a disease of this nature, is henceforward protected against a similar contagion.[*]

It is well known that *retention of urine with ineffectual efforts to urinate,* is one of the most common and painful evils which the use of *cantharides* produces. This point has been sufficiently established by J. Camerarius, Baccius, Van Hilden, Forest, J. Lanzoni, Van der Wiel, and Werlhoff.[†] Cantharides, administered internally, and with precaution, ought, consequently, to be a very salutary homœopathic remedy in similar cases of painful dysury. And this is in reality the case. For, without enumerating all the Greek physicians who, instead of our cantharides, made use of *meloë cichorii,* Fabricius ab Aquapendente, Capo di Vacca, Riedlin, Th. Bartholin,[‡] Young,[§] Smith,[||] Raymond,[**] De Meza,[††] Brisbane,[‡‡] and

---

[*] This mode of homœopathic cure *in antecessum,* (which is called preservation or prophylaxy,) also appears possible in many other cases. For example, by carrying on our persons sulphur, we think we are preserved from the itch which is so common among wool-workers; and by taking as feeble a dose as possible of belladonna, that we are protected from scarlet fever.

[†] See my Fràgmenta de viribus medicamentorum positivis. Leipsic, 1805, i. p. 83.

[‡] Epist. 4, p. 345.

[§] Phil. Trans. No. 280.

[||] Medic. Communications, ii. p. 505.

[**] In Auserlesene Abhandl. für pract. Aerzte. (Select Treatises for Practical Physicians,) iii. p. 460.

[††] Act. Reg. Soc. Med. Hafn. ii. p. 302.

[‡‡] Auserlesene Fälle, (Selected Cases,) Altenburg, 1777.

others, performed perfect cures of very painful ischury that was not dependant upon any mechanical obstacle, with *cantharides.* Huxham has seen this remedy produce the best effects in cases of the same nature; he praises it highly, and would wiillngly have made use of it had not the precepts of the old school of medicine (which, deeming itself wiser than nature herself, prescribes in such cases soothing and relaxing remedies) prevented him, contrary to his own conviction, from using a remedy which, in such cases, is specific or homœopathic.* In cases of recent inflammatory gonorrhea, where Sachs von Lewenheim, Hannæus, Bartholin, Lister, Mead, and chiefly Werlhoff, administered cantharides in very small doses with perfect success, this substance manifestly removed the most severe symptoms which began to declare themselves.†

It produced this effect by virtue of the faculty it possesses (according to the testimony of almost every observer) of exciting painful ischury, urinary heat, inflammation of the urethra, (Wendt,) and even, when applied only externally, a species of inflammatory gonorrhea (Wichman)‡.

The application of sulphur internally very often occasions, in persons of an irritable disposition, *tenesmus,* sometimes even attended with *vomiting* and *griping,* as attested by Walther.§ It is by virtue of this property which sulphur exhibits, that physicians have been able‖ to cure with its aid, dysenteric attacks, and hemorrhoidal diseases attended with tenesmus, as observed by Werlhoff,** and according to Rave,†† hemorrhoidal colics.

* Opera, edit. Reichel, t. ii. p. 124.

† I say " the most severe symptoms which began to declare themselves," because the subsequent treatment demands other considerations; for, although there may have been cases of gonorrhea so slight as to disappear very soon of themselves, and almost without any assistance whatever, still there are others of a graver nature, especially that which is become so common since the time of the French campaigns, which might be called gonorrhea sycotica, and which is communicated by coition, like the chancrous disease, although of a very different nature.

‡ Auswahl aus den Nürnberger gelehrten Unterhaltungen, i. p. 249, note.

§ Progr. de Sulphure et Marte, Lips. 1743, p. 5.

‖ Medic. National-Zeitung, (National Med. Gazette,) 1798, p. 153.

** Observat. de Febribus, p. 3, § 6.

†† In Hufeland's Journal, VII. ii. p 168.

It is well known that the waters at Tœplitz, like all other warm sulphurous mineral waters, frequently excite the appearance of an *exanthema*, which strongly resembles the *itch*, so prevalent among persons employed in *wool-working*. It is precisely this homœopathic virtue which they possess that removes various kinds of psoric eruptions. Can there be any thing more *suffocating* than *sulphurous fumes?* Yet it is the vapour arising from the combustion of sulphur that Bucquet[*] discovered to be the best means of reanimating persons in a state of asphyxia produced by another cause.

From the writings of Beddoes and others, we learn that the English physicians found *nitric acid* of great utility in salivation and ulceration of the mouth, occasioned by the use of mercury. This acid could never have proved useful in such cases, if it did not of itself excite salivation and ulceration of the mouth. To produce these effects, it is only necessary to bathe the surface of the body with it, as Scott[†] and Blair[‡] observe, and the same will occur if administered internally, according to the testimony of Aloyn,[§] Luke,[||] Ferriar,[**] and G. Kelly.[††]

Fritze[‡‡] saw a species of *tetanus* produced by a bath impregnated with *carbonate of potash;* and A. von Humboldt,[§§] by the application of a solution of *salt of tartar* increased the irritability of the muscles to such a degree as to excite tetanic spasm. The curative power which caustic potash exercises in all kinds of tetanus, in which Stütz and others have found it so useful, could it be accounted for in a more simple or rational manner than by the faculty which this alkali possesses of producing homœopathic effects?

---

[*] Edinb. Med. Comment. IX.

[†] In Hufeland's Journal, IV. p. 353.

[‡] Neueste Erfahrungen, (Most Recent Discoveries,) Glogau, 1801.

[§] In the Mémoires de la Soc. Méd. d'Emulation, I. p. 195.

[||] In Beddoes.

[**] In the Sammlung auserles. Abhandl. für Pract. Aertze, (Select Treatises for Practical Physicians, XIX. ii.

[††] Ibid. XIX. i.

[‡‡] In Hufeland's Journal, XII. i. p. 116.

[§§] Versuch über die gereizte Muskel—und Nervenfascr, (Treatise on the Irritability of the Muscles and Nerves,) Posen and Berlin, 1797.

Arsenic, whose effects are so powerful upon the human economy that we cannot decide whether it is more hurtful in the hands of the fool-hardy than it is salutary in those of the wise,—arsenic could never have effected so many remarkable cures of cancer in the face, as witnessed by numerous physicians, among whom I will only cite Fallopius,* Bernhardt,† and Roennow,‡ if this metallic oxide did not possess the homœopathic power of producing, in healthy persons, *very painful tubercles, which are cured with difficulty,* as witnessed by Amatus Lusitanus ;§ very deep and *malignant ulcerations,* according to the testimony of Heinreich|| and Knape ;** and *cancerous ulcers,* as testified by Heinze.†† The ancients would not have been unanimous in the praise which they bestowed on the magnetic arsenical plaster of Angelus Sala‡‡ against pestilential buboes and carbuncles, if arsenic did not, according to the report of Degner§§ and Pfann,|||| give rise to inflammatory tumours which *quickly turn to gangrene,* and to carbuncles or malignant pustules, as observed by Verzascha*** and Pfann.††† And whence could arise that curative power which it exhibits in certain species of intermittent fevers, (a virtue attested by so many thousands of examples, but in the practical application of which, sufficient precaution has not yet been observed, and which virtue was asserted centuries ago by Nicholas Myrepsus, and subsequently placed beyond a doubt by the testimony of Slevogt, Molitor, Jacobi, J. C. Bernhardt, Jüngken, Fauve, Brera, Darwin, May, Jackson, and Fowler,) if it did not proceed from *its peculiar faculty of excit-*

* De Ulceribus et Tumoribus, lib. 2. Venice, 1563.
† In the Journal de Médecine, Chirurg. et Pharm. lvii. March, 1782.
‡ Konigl. Vetensk. Acad. Handl. f. a. 1776.
§ Obs. et Cur. cent. ii. cur. 34.
|| Act. Nat. Cur. ii. obs. 10.
** Annalen der Staatsarzneikunde, I. i.
†† In Hufeland's Journal for September, 1813, p. 48.
‡‡ Anatom. Vitrioli, t. ii. in Opera Med. Chym. Frankfort, 1647, pp. 381, 463.
§§ Act. Nat. Cur. VI.
|||| Annalen der Staatsarzneikunde, loc. cit.
*** Obs. med. cent. Basil, 1677, obs. 66.
††† Samml. Merkwürd. Fälle. (Collection of remarkable cases.) Nuremberg, 1750, pp. 119, 130.

ing fever, as almost every observer of the evils resulting from this substance has remarked, particularly Amatus Lusitanus, Degner, Buchholz, Heun, and Knape.* We may confidently believe E. Alexander,† when he tells us that *arsenic* is a sovereign remedy in some cases of angina pectoris, since Tachenius, Guilbert, Preussius, Thilenius, and Pyl, have seen it give rise to very strong *oppression of the chest;* Gresselius,‡ to a *dyspnœa approaching even to suffocation;* and Majault,§ in particular, saw it produce *sudden attacks of asthma excited by walking, attended with great depression of the vital powers.*

The *convulsions* which are caused by the administration of *copper,* and those observed by Tondi, Ramsay, Fabas, Pyl, and Cosmier, as proceeding from the use of aliments impregnated with copper; the reiterated *attacks of epilepsy,* which J. Lazerme‖ saw result from the accidental introduction of a copper coin into the stomach, and which Pfündel** saw produced by the ingestion of a compound of sal ammoniac and copper into the digestive canal, sufficiently explain, to those physicians who will take the trouble to reflect upon it, how *copper* has been able to cure a case of chorea, as reported by R. Willan,†† Walcker,‡‡ Thesussink,§§ and Delarive,‖‖ and why preparations of copper have so frequently effected the cure of epilepsy, as attested by Batty, Baumes, Bierling, Boerhave, Causland, Cullen, Duncan, Feuerstein, Helvetius, Lieb, Magennis, C. F. Michaelis, Reil, Russel, Stisser, Thilenius, Weissmann, Weizenbreyer, Whithers, and others.

If Poterius, Wepfer, Wedel, F. Hoffman, R. A. Vogel, Thierry, and Albrecht, have cured a species of phthisis, hectic fever, chronic catarrh, and mucous asthma, with *stannum,* it is because this metal possesses the faculty of producing a species

* See my Mat. Med. vol. ii.
† Med. Comm. of Edinb. Dec. t. i. p. 85.
‡ Misc. Nat. Cur. dec. I. ann. 2, p. 149.
§ In the Sammlung Auserles. Abhandl. für Aerzte, VII. 1.
‖ De morbis internis capitis.   Amsterdam, 1748, p. 253.
** In Hufeland's Journal, II. p. 264; and according to the testimony of Burdach, in his System of Medicine, i. Leip. 1807, p. 284.
†† Sammlung Auserles. Abhandl. XII. p. 62.
‡‡ Ibid. XI. iii. p. 672.
§§ Waarnemingen, No. 18.
‖‖ In Kühn's Phys. Med. Journal, January, 1800, p. 58.

of *phthisis*, as Stahl* has observed. And how could it cure *pains of the stomach*, as Geischläger says it does, if it was not capable of exciting a similar malady. Geischläger himself,[†] and Stahl [‡] before him, have proved that it does possess this power.

The evil effects of *lead*, which produces the most *obstinate constipation*, and even the *iliac passion*, (as Thunberg, Wilson, Lazuriaga, and others, inform us,) do they not also give us to understand that this metal possesses likewise the virtue of curing these two affections? Like every other medicine, it ought to subdue and cure, in a permanent manner, the natural diseases which bear a resem' lance to those which it engenders, by reason of the faculty which it possesses of exciting morbid symptoms. Angelus Sala[§] cured a species of ileus, and J. Agricola,[‖] another kind of constipation which endangered the life of the patient, by administering lead internally. The *saturnine* pills with which many physicians (Chirac, Van Helmont, Naudeau, Pererius, Rivinus, Sydenham, Zacutus Lusitanus, Block, and others) cured the iliac passion and obstinate constipation, did not operate merely in a mechanical manner by reason of their weight; for, if such had been the sources of their efficacy, gold, whose weight is greater than that of lead, would have been preferable in such a case; but the pills acted particularly as a saturnine internal remedy, and cured homœopathically. If Otto-Tachenius and Saxtorph formerly cured cases of obstinate hypochondriasis with the aid of *lead*, we ought to bear in mind that this metal tends of itself to excite hypochondriasis, as may be seen in the description of its ill effects given by Lazuriaga.[**]

We ought not to be surprised that Marcus[††] speedily cured an inflammatory swelling of the tongue and of the pharynx with a remedy (*mercury*) which, according to the daily experience of physicians, has a specific tendency to produce *inflammation and tumefaction of the internal parts of the mouth*, phenomena to which it gives rise when merely applied to the

* Mat. Med., cap. 6, p. 83.   † In Hufeland's Journal, X. iii. p. 165.
‡ Mat. Med. loc. cit.   § Opera, p. 213.
‖ Comment. in J. Poppii chym. med. Lips. 1638, p. 223.
** Recueil périod. de Littérature, i. p. 20.
†† Magazin, II. ii.

surface of the body in the form of ointment or plaster, as experienced by Degner,* Friese,† Alberti.‡ Engel,§ and many others. The *weakening of the intellectual faculties*, (Swediaur,‖) *imbecility*, (Degner.**) and *mental alienation*, (Larry,††) which have been seen to result from the use of *mercury*, joined to the almost specific faculty which this metal is known to possess of exciting salivation, explain how W. Perfect‡‡ was enabled, with the use of mercury, to cure in a permanent manner, a case of melancholy alternating with increased secretion of saliva. How does it happen that preparations of mercury proved so successful in the hands of Seelig,§§ in the treatment of angina, accompanied with purpura; in those of Hamilton,‖‖ Hoffman,*** Marcus,††† Rush,‡‡‡ Colden,§§§ Bailey, and Michaelis,‖‖‖ in the treatment of other kinds of malignant quinsy?' It is evidently because this metal brings on of itself a species of angina of the worst description.**** It is certainly by homœopathic means that Sauter†††† cured an ulcerous inflammation of the mouth, accompanied

---

* Act. Nat. Cur. VI. app.

† Geschichte und Versuche einer Chirurg. Gesellschaft. (History and Experiments of a Chirurg. Soc.) Copenhagen, 1774.

‡ Jurisprudentia Medica, V. p. 600.

§ Specimina Medica. Berlin, 1781, p. 99.

‖ Traité des Malad. Vénér. II. p. 368.   ** Loc. cit.

†† Memoirs and Observations in the Description of Egypt, vol. i.

‡‡ Annalen einer Anstalt für Wahnsinnige. (Annals of an Institute for Mad Persons.) Hanover, 1804.

§§ In Hufeland's Journal, XVI. 1, p. 24.

‖‖ Edinb. Med. Comment. IX. 1, p. 8.

*** Medic. Wochenblatt, 1787, No. 1.

††† Magazin für Specielle Therapie, II. p. 334.

‡‡‡ Medic. Inquir. and Observ. No. 6.

§§§ Medic. Observ. and Inquir. 1, No. 19, p. 211.

‖‖‖ In Richter's Chirurg. Biblioth. V. pp. 737—739.

**** Physicians have likewise endeavoured to cure the *croup* by means of mercury; but they generally failed in the attempt, because this metal cannot produce (of itself) in the mucous membrane of the trachea, a change similar to that particular modification which this disease engenders. *Sulphuretem calcis*, which excites cough by impeding respiration, and still more so, the tincture of sponga tosta, act more homœopathically in their special effects, and are consequently much more efficacious, particularly when administered in the *smallest possible doses*. (See my Mat. Med. vi.)

†††† In Hufeland's Journal, VII. ii.

with aphthæ and fœtor of the breath, similar to that which occurs in salivation, when he prescribed a solution of corrosive sublimate as a gargle, and that Block* removed aphthæ by the use of mercurial preparations, since, among other *ulcerations of the mouth*, this substance particularly produces a species of *aphthæ*, as we are informed by Schlegel† and Th. Acrey.‡

Hecker§ used various medicinal compounds successfully in a case of caries succeeding small-pox. Fortunately, a portion of *mercury* was contained in each of these mixtures, to which it may be imagined that this malady will yield (homœopathically) because mercury is one of the few medicinal agents which excites of itself caries, as proved by the many excessive mercurial courses used against syphilis, or even against other diseases, among which are those related by G. P. Michaelis.‖ This metal, which becomes so formidable when its use is prolonged, on account of the caries of which it then becomes the exciting cause, exercises, notwithstanding, a very salutary homœopathic influence in the caries which follows mechanical injuries of the bones, some very remarkable instances of which have been transmitted to us by J. Schlegel,** Joerdens,†† and J. M. Müller.‡‡ The cure of caries (not venereal) of another kind, which has likewise been effected by means of mercury by J. F. G. Neu§§ and J. D. Metzger,‖‖ furnishes a fresh proof of the homœopathic curative virtue with which this substance is endowed.

In perusing the works which have been published on the subject of medical electricity, it is surprising to see what analogy exists between the morbid symptoms sometimes produced by this agent, and the natural diseases which it has cured in a durable manner by homœopathic influence. Innu-

* Medic. Bemerkungen, (Med. Observations,) p. 161.
† In Hufeland's Journal, VII. iv.
‡ London Med. Journal, 1788.
§ In Hufeland's Journal, i. p. 362.
‖ Ibid. June, 1809, vi. p. 57.
** Hufeland's Journal, v. pp. 605, 610.
†† Ibid. X. ii.
‡‡ Obs. Med. Chirur. ii. cas. 10.
§§ Diss. Med. Pract. Goettingæ, 1776.
‖‖ Adversaria, p. ii. sect. 4.

merable are the authors who have observed that *acceleration of the pulse* is among the first effects of positive electricity; but Sauvages,[*] Delas,[†] and Barillon,[‡] have seen *febrile paroxysms* excited by *electricity.* The faculty it has of *producing fever,* is the cause to which we may attribute the circumstance of Gardini,[§] Wilkinson,[||] Syme,[**] and Wesley,[††] curing with it alone tertian fever, and likewise the removal of quartan fevers by Zetzel[‡‡] and Willermoz.[§§] It is also known that electricity occasions a contraction of the muscles which resembles a *convulsive movement.* De Sans[||||] was enabled to excite even *continued convulsions* in the arm of a young girl as often as he pleased to make the experiment. It is by virtue of this power which electricity develops, that De Sans[***] and Franklin[†††] applied it successfully in convulsions, and that Theden[‡‡‡] cured with its aid a little girl ten years of age who lost her speech and partially the use of her left arm by lightning, yet kept up a constant involuntary movement of the arms and legs, accompanied by a spasmodic contraction of the fingers of the left hand. Electricity likewise produced a kind of ischias, as observed by Jallobert[§§§] and another;[||||||] it has also cured this affection by similarity of effect, (homœopathically,) as confirmed by Hiortberg, Lovet, Arrigoni, Daboueix, Manduyt, Symè, and Wesley. Several physicians have cured a species of ophthalmia by electricity, that is to say, by means of the power which it has of exciting of itself *inflammation of the eyes,* as observed by P. Dickson[****] and Bertholon.[††††] Finally, it has in the hands of Fushel cured varices; and it owes this sanative virtue to the faculty which Jallobert[‡‡‡‡] ascribes to it of producing *varicose tumours.*

---

[*] In Bertholon de St. Lazare, Medicinische Electrisität, von Kühn. (Medical Electricity.) Leip. 1788, t. i. pp. 239, 240.

[†] Ibid. p. 232.   [‡] Ibid. p. 233.   [§] Ibid. p. 232.

[||] Ibid. p. 251.   [**] Ibid. p. 250.   [††] Ibid. p. 249.

[‡‡] Ibid. p. 52.   [§§] Ibid. p. 250.   [||||] Ibid p. 274.

[***] Ibid. p. 274.   [†††] Recueil sur l'Electr. Medic. ii. p. 386.

[‡‡‡] Neue Bemerkungen und Erfahrungen, iii. (Recent Observations and Experiments.)

[§§§] Expériences et Observations sur l'Electricité.

[||||||] Philos. Trans. vol. 63.   [****] Bertholon, loc. cit. p. 406.

[††††] Loc. cit. ii. p. 296.   [‡‡‡‡] Loc. cit.

Albers relates, that a warm bath at one hundred degrees of the thermometer of Fahrenheit greatly reduced the burning of an acute fever, in which the pulse beat one hundred and thirty to the minute, and that it brought back the pulsation to the number of one hundred and ten. Löffler found hot fomentations very useful in encephalitis occasioned by insulation or the action of the heat of stoves,* and Callisen† regards affusions of warm water on the head as the most efficacious of all remedies in cases of inflammation of the brain.

If we except those cases where ordinary physicians have discovered (not by their own research but by *vulgar empiricism*) the specific remedy for a disease which always retained its identity, and by whose aid they could consequently cure it in a direct manner; such, for example, as mercury in the chancrous venereal disease, arnica in a malady resulting from contusions, cinchona in intermittent fevers arising from marsh miasmata, sulphur in a recent development of itch, &c.;—I say, if we except all these cases, we shall find that those which they have cured promptly and permanently by the bounty of Providence alone, are to the mass of their other irrational cures in the proportion of one to a thousand.

Sometimes they were conducted by mere chance to a homœopathic mode of treatment ;‡ but yet they did not perceive the

* In Hufeland's Journal, iii. p. 630.
† Act. Soc. Med. Hafn. iv. p. 419.
‡ Thus, for example, they always imagine they can drive out the perspiration through the skin (which they say stops up the pores after catching cold) by administering, in the cold stage of the fever, an infusion of the flowers of the sambucus niger, which is capable of subduing such fevers homœopathically, and restores the patient to health. The cure is most effectually and speedily performed, without transpiration, when the patient drinks but little of this liquor and abstains from all other medicines. They often apply repeated warm cataplasms to acute tumours whose excessive inflammation, attended with insupportable pain, prevents suppuration taking place. Under the influence of this treatment the inflammation soon diminishes, the pain decreases, and the abscess is quickly formed, as may be discovered by the fluctuation and appearance of the surface. They imagine that they have

law of nature by which cures of this kind are and ever must be performed.

It is therefore highly important to the welfare of the human race, that we should examine how these cures, which are as remarkable for their rare occurrence as they are surprising in their effects, are performed. The result is one of the deepest interest. The examples which we have cited, sufficiently prove, that these cures have never taken place but by homœopathic means, that is to say, by the faculty of exciting a morbid state similar to the disease that was to be cured. They have been performed in a prompt and permanent manner by medicines, upon which, those who prescribed them (contrary to all the existing systems of therapeutics) have fallen as it were by chance, without well knowing what they were doing or why they acted in this manner. Contrary to their inclinations,

softened the tumour by the moisture of the cataplasm, while they have done nothing more than. destroy the excess of inflammation homœopathically by the stronger heat of the cataplasm, and promoted suppuration. Why is the red oxide of mercury (which forms the basis of the ointment of St. Ives) of such utility in certain cases of ophthalmia, when of all substances there is none more capable of producing inflammation of the eyes? It is difficult to perceive that in this case its action is homœopathic? How could the juice of parsley procure instantaneous relief in cases of dysury so frequent among children, or in ordinary cases of gonorrhea, which are principally distinguished by painful and vain attempts to pass water, if this juice did not cure homœopathically by the faculty which it possesses of exciting painful dysury in healthy persons? The saxifrage, which excites an abundant mucous secretion in the bronchiæ and pharynx, is a salutary remedy for the so-called mucous angina; and certain kinds of uterine hemorrhage are stopped by small doses of the leaves of sabina, which has the property of exciting metrorrhagia: in both instances these remedies are applied without any knowledge of the therapeutic law of homœopathy. Opium, which produces costiveness, has been found, in small doses, to be one of the principal and most certain remedies in constipation from incarcerated hernia and ileus, without ever leading to a discovery of the homœopathic law which is evident in such cases. Ulcers in the throat (not venereal) have been cured homœopathically by small doses of mercury. Diarrhœa has frequently been stopped by the use of rhubarb, which produces alvine evacuations; rabies has been removed by means of belladonna, which excites a species of hydrophobia; and finally, coma, which is so dangerous in acute fevers, has been cured, as if by enchantment, by a small dose of opium, a substance which occasions heat and stupefaction. And after all these examples, which speak loudly for themselves, there are still physicians who repulse homœopathy with disdain!

they by this fact confirmed the necessity of the sole law of nature in therapeutics, that of homœopathy; a law, which *medical* prejudices, till now, would not permit us to search after, notwithstanding the infinite number of facts and visible signs which ought to have pointed towards its discovery.

Even in the practice of domestic medicine by persons ignorant of our profession, but who were gifted with sound judgment and discerning minds, it was discovered that the homœopathic method of cure was the safest, the most rational, and the least subject to failure.

Frozen sourcrout is frequently applied to a limb that is recently frozen, or sometimes it is rubbed with snow.

A cook who has scalded his hand, exposes it to the fire at a certain distance, without heeding the increase of pain which it at first occasions, because experience has taught him that by acting thus, he can in a very short time perfectly cure the burn, and remove every feeling of pain.*

Other intelligent individuals, equally strangers to medical science—such, for example, as the lacker-workers, apply a substance to burns which excites of itself a similar feeling of *heat*, that is to say, hot *alcohol* or the *oil of turpentine*,† and by

---

* Fernel (in his Therapeutics, book vi. cap. 20,) considered that the best means to allay pain, was to expose the part that was burnt to the fire. John Hunter (in his work on the blood, p. 218) mentions the great inconvenience that results from the application of cold water to burns, and prefers the method of exposing the parts to the fire. In this he departs from the traditional doctrines of medicine, which prescribe cooling remedies in cases of inflammation (*contraria contrariis*) ; but experience proved to him that a homœopathic heat (*similia similibus*) would be most salutary.

† Sydenham (Opera, p. 271) says that repeated applications of *alcohol* are preferable to all other remedies in burns. B. Bell (System of Surgery, 1789) expresses himself equally favourable with regard to the efficacy of homœopathic remedies. These are his words: "*Alcohol* is one of the best remedies for burns of every description : on the first application it appears to increase the pain, (see § 160,) but the latter is soon allayed, and gives place to an agreeable sensation of calm and tranquillity. This method is never more efficacious than when the whole part is plunged into alcohol ; but where the immersion is not practicable, it is requisite to keep the burn continually covered with pledgets imbibed with this liquid." I further add, *that warm, and even very hot alcohol, affords still more prompt and certain relief, because it is far more homœopathic than alcohol that is cold.* This is confirmed by every experience.

Edward Kentish treated several men who were often dreadfully burned in

7

these means cure themselves in a few hours, well knowing that the so-called cooling ointments would not produce the same result in an equal number of months, and that cold water* would only make the evil worse.

the coal mines by the explosion of fire-damp; he made them apply hot oil of turpentine or alcohol, as being the best remedies that could be used in severe burns. (Second Essay on Burns, London, 1798.) No treatment is more homœopathic than this, nor can there be any more efficacious. The worthy and skilful physician, Heister, also recommends this practice from his own personal experience, (Instit. Chirurg. Tom. I. p 333); he praises the application of the oil of turpentine, of alcohol, and of cataplasms as hot as the patient can bear them. But nothing can more strongly exhibit the surprising superiority of the homœopathic method (that is to say of the application of substances that excite a sensation of heat and burning, to parts that are burned) over the palliative, (which consists of cold applications,) than those simple experiments where, in order to compare the results of these two opposite proceedings, they have been simultaneously tried upon the same patient, and on parts that were burned in an equal degree. Thus J. Bell, (Kühn's Phys. Med. Journal for June, 1801, p. 428,) having to treat a lady who had scalded both arms with boiling liquid, covered one with the oil of *turpentine*, and plunged the other into *cold water*. The first was no longer painful at the expiration of half an hour, while the other continued so during six hours: the moment it was withdrawn from the cold water the patient *experienced far greater pain, and it required much longer time to cure this arm than it did to heal the other.* J. Anderson (Kentish, loc. cit. p. 43) likewise treated a woman who had scalded her face and arm with boiling fat. "The face, which was very red and painful, was covered with oil of turpentine a few minutes after the accident: as for the arm, the patient had already plunged it of her own accord into cold water, and expressed a desire to await the result of this treatment for a few hours. At the expiration of seven hours the face was better, and the patient relieved in this part. With regard to the arm, around which the water had been several times renewed, it became exceedingly painful whenever it was withdrawn from the water, and the inflammation had manifestly increased. The next day I found that the patient had suffered extreme pain in the arm; inflammation had extended above the elbow, several large blisters had burst, and a thick eschar had formed itself upon the arm and hand, which were then covered with a warm cataplasm. The face was no longer painful, but it was necessary to apply emollients a fortnight longer to cure the arm." *Who does not perceive, in this instance, the great superiority of the homœopathic mode of treatment, (that is to say, of the application of agents which produce effects resembling the evil itself,) over the antipathic prescribed by the ordinary physicians of the old school of medicine?*

* J. Hunter is not the only one who has pointed out the evil results that attend the treatment of burns with cold water. Fabricius de Hilden, (De

An experienced reaper, however little he may be accustomed to the use of strong liquors, will not drink cold water (contraria contrariis) when the heat of the sun or the fatigue of hard labour have brought him into a feverish state : he is well aware of the danger that would ensue, and therefore takes a small quantity of some heating liquor—viz. a mouthful of brandy. Experience, the source of all truth, has convinced him of the advantage and efficacy of this homœopathic mode of proceeding. The heat and lassitude which oppressed him, soon diminish.*

Occasionally there have been certain physicians who guessed that medicines might cure diseases by the faculty which they possessed of exciting morbid symptoms that resembled the disease itself.†

Thus the author of the book περὶ τόπων τῶν κατ' ἄνθρωπον,‡ which forms a part of the works attributed to Hippocrates, expresses himself in the following remarkable words: διὰ τὰ ὅμοια νοῦσος γίνεται, καὶ διὰ τὰ ὅμοια προσφερόμενα ἐκ νοσεόντων ὑγιαίνονται, —διὰ τὸ ἐμέειν ἔμετος παύεται.

Physicians of a later period have likewise known and proclaimed the truths of homœopathy. Thus *B. Boulduc*,§ for

---

Combustionibus Libellus. Basil, 1607, cap. V. p. 11,) likewise assures us that cold applications are very hurtful in such cases, that they produce the most disastrous effects—that inflammation, suppuration, and sometimes gangrene, are the consequences.

* Zimmerman (Ueber die Erfahrung, II. p. 318,) tells us that the inhabitants of warm countries act in the same manner, with the most beneficial results, and that they usually drink a small quantity of spirituous liquors when they are much heated.

† In citing the following passages of writers who have had some presentiment of homœopathy, I do not mean to prove the excellence of the method, (which establishes itself without further proof,) but I wish to free myself from a reproach of having passed them over in silence to arrogate to myself the merit of the discovery.

‡ Basil, Froben, 1538, p. 72.

§ Mém. de l'Acad. Royale, 1710.

example, discovered that the purgative properties of rhubarb were the faculty by which this plant cured diarrhœa.

Detharding guessed[*] that the infusion of senna would cure the colic in adults by virtue of the faculty which it possesses of exciting that malady in healthy persons.

Bertholon[†] informs us, that in diseases electricity diminishes and finally removes a pain which is very similar to one which it also produces.

Thoury[‡] affirms that positive electricity accelerates arterial pulsation, also that it renders the same slower where it is already quickened by disease.

Stoerck[§] was struck with the idea, that if stramonium disturbs the senses and produces mental derangement in persons who are healthy, it might very easily be administered to maniacs for the purpose of restoring the senses by effecting a change of ideas.

The Danish physician, *Stahl*,[||] has, above all other writers, expressed his conviction on this head most unequivocally. He speaks in the following terms :—"The received method in medicine, of treating diseases by opposite remedies—that is to say, by medicines which are opposed to the effects they produce (*contraria contrariis*),—is completely false and absurd. I am convinced, on the contrary, that diseases are subdued by agents which produce a similar affection, (*similia similibus*) :—burns, by the heat of a fire to which the parts are exposed ; the frost-bite, by snow or icy cold water ; and inflammation and contusions, by spirituous applications. It is by these means I have succeeded in curing a disposition to acidity of the stomach, by using very small doses of sulphuric acid in cases where a multitude of absorbing powders had been administered to no purpose."

Thus far the great truth has more than once been approached by physicians. But a transitory idea was all that

---

[*] Eph. Nat. Cur. cent. x. obs. 76.
[†] Medic. Electricit. II. pp. 15, 282.
[‡] Mém. lu à l'Acad. de Caen.
[§] Libell. de Stramon. p. 8.
[||] In J. Hummel, Comment. de Arthritide tam tartarea, quam scorbutica, seu podagra et scorbutico. Budingæ, 1738—in 8, pp. 40, 42.

presented itself to them; consequently, the indispensable reform which ought to have taken place in the old school of therapeutics to make room for the true curative method and a system of medicine at once simple and certain, has, till the present day, not been effected.

ORGANON OF MEDICINE.

The sole duty of a physician is, to restore health in a mild, prompt, and durable manner.

§ 1.   The first and *sole* duty of the physician is, to restore health to the sick.*   This is the true art of healing.

* His mission is not, as many physicians (who wasting their time and powers in the pursuit of fame) have imagined it to be, that of inventing systems by stringing together empty ideas and hypotheses upon the immediate essence of life and the origin of disease in the interior of the human economy; nor is it that of continually endeavouring to account for the morbid phenomena with their nearest cause (which must forever remain concealed) and confounding the whole in unintelligible words and pompous observations which make a deep impression on the minds of the ignorant, while the patients are left to sigh in vain for relief.   We have already too many of these learned reveries which bear the name of medical theories, and for the inculcation of which, even special professorships have been established.   It is high time that all those who call themselves physicians should cease to deceive suffering humanity with words that have no meaning, and begin to act—that is to say, to afford relief, and cure the sick in reality.

§ 2.   The perfection of a cure consists in restoring health in a prompt, mild, and permanent manner; in removing and annihilating disease by the shortest, safest, and most certain means, upon principles that are at once plain and intelligible.

The physician ought to search after that which is to be cured in disease, and be acquainted with the curative virtues of medicines, in order to adapt the medicine to the disease.   He must also be acquainted with the means of preserving health.

§ 3.   When the physician clearly perceives the *curative indication* in each particular case of disease—when he is acquainted with the *therapeutic effects of medicines* individually—when, guided by evident reasons, he knows how to make such an application of that which is curative in medicine to that which is indubitably diseased in the patient (both in regard to the choice of the substances, the precise dose to be administered, and the time of repeating it) that a cure may necessarily follow—and finally when he knows what are the obstacles to the cure, and can render the latter permanent by removing them ;—*then only can he accomplish his purpose in a rational manner—then only can he merit the title of a genuine physician, or a man skilled in the art of healing.*

§ 4. The physician is likewise the guardian of health when he knows what are the objects that disturb it, which produce and keep up disease, and can remove them from persons who are in health.

In the cure of disease, it is necessary to regard the fundamental cause, and other circumstances.

§ 5. When a cure is to be performed, the physician must avail himself of all the particulars he can learn, both respecting the probable *origin* of the acute malady and the most significant points in the history of the chronic disease, to aid him in the discovery of their *fundamental cause*, which is commonly due to some chronic miasm. In all researches of this nature, he must take into consideration the apparent state of the physical constitution of the patient, (particularly when the affection is chronic,) the disposition, occupation, mode of life, habits, social relations, age, sexual functions, etc. etc.

For the physician, the totality of the symptoms alone constitutes the disease.

§ 6. The unprejudiced observer, (however great may be his powers of penetration,) aware of the futility of all elaborate speculations that are not confirmed by experience, perceives in each individual affection nothing, but changes of the state of the body and mind, (*traces of disease, casualties, symptoms,*) that are discoverable by the senses alone,—that is to say, deviations from the former sound state of health, which are felt by the patient himself, remarked by the individuals around him, and observed by the physician. The *ensemble* of these available signs represents, in its full extent, the disease itself—that is, they constitute the true and only form of it which the mind is capable of conceiving.*

* I cannot, therefore, comprehend how it was possible for physicians, without heeding the symptoms or taking them as a guide in the treatment, to imagine that they ought to search the interior of the human economy,

(which is inaccessible and concealed from our view,) and that they could there alone discover that which was to be cured in disease. I cannot conceive how they could entertain so ridiculous a pretension as that of being able to discover the internal invisible change that had taken place, and restore the same to the order of its normal condition by the aid of medicines, without ever troubling themselves very much about the symptoms, and that they should have regarded such a method as the only means of performing a radical and rational cure. Is not that which manifests itself in disease, by symptoms, identified with the change itself which has taken place in the human economy, and which it is impossible to discover without their aid? Do not the symptoms of disease, which are sensibly cognizable, represent to the physician the disease itself? When he can neither see the spiritual essence, the vital power which produces the disease, nor yet the disease itself, but simply perceive and learn its morbid effects, that he may be able to treat it accordingly? What would the old school search out farther from the hidden interior for a prima causa morbi, whilst they reject and superciliously despise the palpable and intelligible representation of the disease, the symptoms which clearly announce themselves to us as the object of cure? What is there besides these in disease which they have to cure?**

** The physician who engages in a search after the hidden springs of the internal economy will hourly be deceived; but the homœopathist, who with due attention seizes upon the faithful image of the entire group of symptoms, possesses himself of a guide that may be depended on; and when he has succeeded in destroying the whole of them, he may be certain that he has likewise annihilated the internal and hidden cause of disease." *Rau,* loc. cit. p. 103.

To cure disease, it is merely requisite to remove the entire symptoms, duly regarding, at the same time, the circumstances enumerated in § 5.

§ 7. As in a disease where no manifest or exciting cause presents itself for removal, (*causa occasionalis*,[1]) we can perceive nothing but the symptoms, then must these symptoms alone (with due attention to the accessory circumstances, and the possibility of the existence of a miasm) (§ 5) guide the physician in the choice of a fit remedy to combat the disease. The totality of the symptoms, *this image of the immediate essence of the malady reflected externally,* ought to be the principal or sole object by which the latter could make known the medicines it stands in need of—the only agent to determine the choice of a remedy that would be most appropriate. In short, the *ensemble*[2] of the symptoms is the principal and sole object that a physician ought to have in view in every case of disease—the power of his art is to be directed against that alone in order to cure and transform it into health.

[1] It is taken for granted that every intelligent physician will commence by removing this *causa occasionalis;* then the indisposition usually yields of

itself. Thus it is necessary to remove flowers from the room when their odours occasion paroxysms of fainting and hysteria, to extract from the eye the foreign substance which occasions ophthalmia ; remove the tight bandages from a wounded limb which threatens gangrene, and apply others more suitable ; lay bare and tie up a wounded artery where hemorrhage produces fainting ; evacuate the berries of belladonna, &c., which may have been swallowed, by vomiting ; extract the foreign particles which have introduced themselves into the openings of the body, (the nose, pharynx, ears, urethra, rectum, vagina) ; grind down a stone in the bladder; open the imperforate anus of the new-born infant, &c.

2 Not knowing at times what plan to adopt in disease, physicians ·have till now endeavoured to suppress or annihilate some one of the various symptoms which appeared. This method, which is known by the name of the *symptomatic*, has very justly excited universal contempt, not only because no advantage is derived from it, but because it gives rise to many bad consequences. A single existing symptom is no more the disease itself, than a single leg constitutes the entire of the human body. This method is so much the more hurtful in its effects, that in attacking an isolated symptom, they make use solely of an opposite remedy, (that is to say, of antipathics or palliatives,) so that after an amendment of short duration, the evil bursts forth again worse than before.

When all the symptoms are extinguished, the disease is at the same time internally cured.

§ 8. It is not possible to conceive or prove by any experience, after the cure of the whole of the symptoms of a disease, together with all its perceptible changes, that there remains or possibly can remain any other than a healthy state, or that the morbid alteration which has taken place in the interior of the economy has not been annihilated.*

* In one who has thus been restored from sickness by a genuine physician, so that no trace of disease, no morbid symptom any longer remains, and every token of health has again durably returned, can it for a moment be supposed, without offering an insult to common sense, that the entire corporeal disease still resides in such an individual? and yet Hufeland, at the head of the old school, makes this identical assertion (in his work on Homœopathy, p. 27, l. 19) in the following words, viz., "The homœopathist may remove the symptoms, but the disease will still remain." He affirms this partly out of mortification at the progress and salutary effects of homœopathy, and partly because he entertains wholly *material* ideas of disease, which he is unable to regard as an immaterial change in the organism, produced by the morbid derangement of the vital power ; he does not consider it as a changed condition of the organism, but as a *material something*, which, after the cure is completed, may yet continue to lurk in some internal corner of the body, in order one day or other, at pleasure, and during a period of blooming health, once more to burst forth with its material presence ! So shocking is still the delusion of the

old pathology! That such a one only could produce a *therapeutica*, solely intent upon cleansing out the poor patient, is not surprising.

During health, the system is animated by a spiritual, self-moved, vital power, which preserves it in harmonious order.

§ 9.   In the healthy condition of man, the immaterial vital principle which animates the material body, exercises an absolute sway and maintains all its parts in the most admirable order and harmony, both of sensation and action, so that our indwelling rational spirit may freely employ these living, healthy organs for the superior purposes of our existence.

Without this vital, dynamic power, the organism is dead.

§ 10.   The material organism deprived of its vital principle, is incapable of sensation, action, or self-preservation ;* it is the immaterial vital principle only, animating the former in its healthy and morbid condition, that imparts to it all sensation, and enables it to perform its functions.

* It is then dead, and subjected to the physical laws of the external world ; it suffers decay, and is again resolved into its constituent elements.

In disease, the vital power only is primarily disturbed, and expresses its sufferings (internal changes) by abnormal alterations in the sensations and actions of the system.

§ 11.   In disease, this spontaneous and immaterial vital principle pervading the physical organism, is primarily deranged by the dynamic influence of a morbific agent which is inimical to life.   Only the vital principle thus disturbed, can give to the organism its abnormal sensations, and incline it to the irregular actions which we call disease ; for as an invisible principle only cognizable through its operations in the organism, its morbid disturbances can be perceived solely by means of the expression of disease in the sensations and actions of that side of the organism exposed to the senses of the physician and bystanders ; in other words, by the *morbid symptoms*, and can be indicated in no other manner.

By the extinction of the totality of the symptoms in the process of cure, the suffering of the vital power, that is, the entire morbid affection, inwardly and outwardly, is removed.

§ 12.   It is solely the morbidly affected vital principle which brings forth diseases,* so that the expression of disease, perceptible by the senses, announces at the same time all the internal change, that is, all the morbid perturbations of the vital principle; in short, it displays the entire disease. Consequently, after a cure is effected, the cessation of all morbid expression, and of all sensible changes which are inconsistent with the healthy performance of the functions, necessarily pre-supposes, with an equal degree of certainty, a restoration of the vital principle to its state of integrity and the recovered health of the whole organism.

* In what manner the vital principle produces morbid indications in the system, that is, *how* it produces disease, is to the physician a useless question, and therefore will ever remain unanswered. Only that which is necessary for him to know of the disease, and which is fully sufficient for the purpose of cure, has the Lord of life rendered evident to his senses.

To presume that disease (non-chirurgical) is a peculiar and distinct something, residing in man, is a conceit which has rendered allœopathy so pernicious.

§ 13. Disease, therefore, (those forms of it not belonging to manual surgery,) considered as it is by the allœopathists as *something* separate from the living organism and the vital principle which animates it, as something hidden internally, and material, how subtile soever its nature may be supposed, is a non-entity, which could only be conceived in heads of material mould, and which for ages, hitherto, has given to medicine all those pernicious deviations which constitute it a mischievous art.

Every curable disease is made known to the physician by its symptoms.

§ 14. There is no curable malady, nor any invisible morbid change, in the interior of man, which admits of cure, that is not made known by morbid indications or symptoms to the physician of accurate observation—a provision entirely in conformity with the infinite goodness of the all-wise Preserver of men.

The sufferings of the deranged vital power, and the morbid symptoms produced thereby, as an invisible whole, one and the same.

§ 15. The sufferings of the immaterial vital principle which animates the interior of our bodies, when it is morbidly disturbed, and the mass of symptoms produced by it in the or-

ganism, which are externally manifested, and represent the
actual malady, constitute a whole—they are one and the
same. The organism is, indeed, the material instrument of
life; but without that animation which is derived from the
instinctive sensibility and control of the vital principle, its existence is as inconceivable as that of a vital principle without
an organism; consequently, both constitute a unit—although,
for the sake of ease in comprehension, our minds may separate
this unity into two ideas.

*It is only by means of the spiritual influence of a morbific agent, that our
spiritual vital power can be diseased; and in like manner, only by the
spiritual (dynamic) operation of medicine, that health can be restored.*

§ 16. By the operation of injurious influences, from without, upon the healthy organism, influences which disturb the
harmonious play of the functions, the vital principle, as a
spiritual dynamis, cannot otherwise be assailed and affected
than in a (dynamic) spiritual manner; neither can such morbid disturbances, or in other words, such diseases, be removed
by the physician, except in like manner, by means of the
spiritual (dynamic virtual) countervailing agency of the suitable medicines acting upon the same vital principle, and this
action is communicated by the sentient nerves everywhere
distributed in the organism; so that curative medicines possess the faculty of restoring, and do actually restore health,
with concomitant functional harmony, by a dynamic influence
only, acting upon the vital energies, after the morbid alterations in the health of the patient which are evident to the
senses (the totality of the symptoms) have represented the
disease to the attentive and observant physician as fully as
may be requisite to effect a cure.

*The physician has only to remove the totality of the symptoms, and he has
cured the entire disease.*

§ 17. As the cure which is effected by the annihilation of
all the symptoms of a disease removes at the same time the
internal change upon which the disease is founded—that is to
say, destroys it in its totality[1]—it is accordingly clear, that the
physician has nothing more to do than destroy the totality
of the symptoms in order to effect a simultaneous removal of

the internal change—that is, to annihilate the *disease itself.*
But by destroying disease we restore health, the first r nd sole
duty of the physician who is sensible of the importance of his
calling, which consists in affording relief to his fellow mortals,
and not in discoursing dogmatically.[2]

[1] A dream, a presentiment resulting from a superstitious imagination, a
solemn prediction, impressing a person with the belief that he will infallibly
die on a certain day and at a certain hour, have often produced the embryo of
the growing disease, the signs of approaching death, and even death itself at
the hour prognosticated. Such effects could never take place without some
change having been operated in the interior of the body, corresponding with
the state which manifested itself externally. In cases of this nature, it has
also sometimes happened, that by deceiving the patient or insinuating a contrary belief, it has succeeded in dissipating all the morbid appearances which
announced the approach of death, and suddenly restored him to health : circumstances that never could have taken place without annihilating at the
same time, by this moral remedy, the internal morbid change of which death
was to be the result.

[2] The wisdom and goodness of the Creator in the cure of disease to which
man is subject, could not be more manifest than in developing to the physician the incidents, in the malady to be removed, openly to the observation of
the physician in order for their removal and the consequent restoration of
health. But what would be thought of those divine attributes if (as the prevalent school of medicine, hitherto affecting a supernatural insight of the
internal nature of things, have pretended) he had veiled what is to be cured
in disease in mystic darkness, wrapt it in concealment within, and thus rendered it impossible for man to know distinctly the malady, and the cure
equally impossible.

The totality of the symptoms is the sole indication in the choice of the remedy.

§ 18. From this incontrovertible truth, that beyond the
totality of the symptoms there is nothing discoverable in diseases by which they could make known the nature of the
medicines they stand in need of, we ought naturally to conclude that there can be *no other indication* whatever than the
ensemble of the symptoms in each individual case to guide us
in the choice of a remedy.

*Changes in the general state, in disease, (symptoms of disease,) can be cured
in no other way, by medicines, than in so far as the latter possess the power,
likewise, of affecting changes in the system.*

§ 19. As *diseases* are nothing more than *changes in the
general state of the human economy* which declare themselves
by symptoms, and the cure being impossible except by the

conversion of the diseased state into one of health, it may be
readily conceived that *medicines* could never cure disease if
they did not possess the faculty of changing the general state
of the system, which consists of sensation and action, and that
their curative virtues are owing to this faculty *alone*.

*This faculty which medicines have of producing changes in the system, can
only be known by observing their effects upon healthy individuals.*

§ 20.   By a mere effort of the mind we could never discover
this innate and hidden *faculty* of medicines—this spiritual
virtue by which they can modify the state of the human body
and even cure disease.   It is by experience only, and observation of the effects produced by their influence on the general
state of the economy, that we can either discover or form to
ourselves any clear conception of it.

*The morbid symptoms which medicines produce in healthy persons are the
sole indications of their curative virtues in disease.*

§ 21.   The curative powers of medicines being nowise discoverable in themselves, a fact which few will venture to dispute, and the pure experiments which have been made even
by the most skilful observers not exhibiting anything to our
view which could be capable of rendering them medicines or
curative remedies, except the faculty which they possess of
producing manifest changes in the general state of the human
economy, particularly with *persons in health*, in whom they
excite morbid symptoms of a very decided character ; we
ought to conclude from this, that when medicines act as remedies, they cannot exercise their curative virtue but by the
faculty which they possess of modifying the general state of
the economy, and giving birth to peculiar symptoms.   Consequently, we ought to rely solely upon the morbid appearances
which medicines excite in healthy persons, the only possible
manifestation of the curative virtues which they possess, in
order to learn what malady each of them produces individually, and at the same time what diseases they are capable
of curin .

*If experience prove that the medicines which produce symptoms similar to
those of the disease, are the therapeutic agents that cure it in the most
certain and permanent manner, we ought to select these medicines in the
cure of the disease.   If, on the contrary, it proves that the most certain*

and permanent cure is obtained by medicinal substances that produce symptoms directly opposite to those of the disease, then the latter agents ought to be selected for this purpose.

§ 22. But, as we can discover nothing to remove in disease in order to change it into health, except the *ensemble* of the symptoms ; as we also perceive nothing curative in medicines but their faculty of producing morbid symptoms in persons who are healthy, and of removing them from those who are diseased, it very naturally follows that medicines assume the character of remedies, and become capable of annihilating disease in no other manner than by exciting particular appearances and symptoms ; or to express it more clearly, a certain artificial disease which destroys the previous symptoms—that is to say, the natural disease which they intend to cure. On the other hand, if we wish to destroy the entire symptoms of a disease, we ought to choose a medicine which has a tendency to excite similar or opposite symptoms, according to that which experience may point out to us as the easiest, safest, and most permanent means of removing the symptoms of the disease, and of restoring health, whether it be by opposing to the latter medicinal symptoms that are similar, or contrary.*

 * Besides these two, there is no other mode of applying medicines in disease but the allœopathic ; and in this latter, remedies are administered which produce symptoms that bear no reference whatever to those of the disease itself, being neither similar nor contrary, but wholly heterogeneous. I have already shown, in the INTRODUCTION, *that this method is an imperfect imitation of the still more imperfect attempts made by the unintelligent vital powers (when abandoned to their own resources) to save themselves at all hazards,* a power to which the organism was confided merely to preserve its harmony so long as health continued. However inapplicable this method may be, it has for so long a time been practised by the existing school of medicine, that the physician can no more pass over it unnoticed, than the historian can be silent on the oppression to which mankind has been subject for thousands of years beneath the absurd rule of despotic governments.

Morbid symptoms that are inveterate cannot be cured by medicinal symptoms of an opposite character (antipathic method).

§ 23. From pure experience and the most careful experiments that have been tried, we learn that the existing morbid symptoms, far from being effaced or destroyed by contrary medicinal symptoms like those excited by the antipathic, enantiopathic, or palliative methods, they, on the contrary, re-appear more intense than ever, after having for a short space of time undergone apparent amendment. (Vide § 58 —62, and 69.)

The homœopathic method, or that which employs medicines producing symptoms similar to those of the malady, is the only one of which experience proves the certain efficacy.

§ 24. There remains, accordingly, no other method of applying medicines profitably in diseases than the homœopathic, by means of which we select from all others that medicine (in order to direct it against the entire symptoms of the individual morbid case) whose manner of acting upon persons in health is known, and which has the power of producing an artificial malady the nearest in resemblance to the natural disease before our eyes.

§ 25. Plain experience,* an infallible oracle in the art of healing, proves to us, in every careful experiment, that the particular medicine whose action upon persons in health produces the greatest number of symptoms resembling those of the disease which it is intended to cure, possesses, also, in reality, (when administered in convenient doses,) the power of suppressing, in a radical, prompt, and permanent manner, the totality of these morbid symptoms—that is to say, (§ 6— 16,) the whole of the existing disease ; it also teaches us that all medicines cure the diseases whose symptoms approach nearest to their own, and that among the latter none admit of exception.

* I do not mean that kind of experience acquired by our ordinary practitioners after having long combated, with a heap of complicated prescriptions, a multitude of diseases which they never examined with care, and which (true to the errors of the old school) they regarded as being already included in our pathology, thinking that they perceived in them some imaginary morbific principle, or some internal anomaly not less hypothetical. In fact, they were in the habit of seeing something, but they knew not what they saw, and they arrived at conclusions which a deity alone could unravel in the midst of so great a concourse of diverse powers acting upon an unknown subject, a result from which no information was to be gained. Fifty years of such experience are like fifty years passed in looking through a kaleidoscope, which, full of unknown things of varied colours, revolves continually upon itself : there would be seen thousands of figures changing their forms every instant without a possibility of accounting for any one of them.

8

This is grounded upon the therapeutic law of nature, that a weaker dynamic affection in man is permanently extinguished by one that is similar, of greater intensity, yet of a different origin.

§ 26.   This phenomenon is founded on the natural law of homœopathy—a law unknown till the present time, although it has on all occasions formed the basis of every visible cure— that is to say, *a dynamic disease in the living economy of man is extinguished in a permanent manner by another that is more powerful, when the latter (without being of the same species) bears a strong resemblance to it in its mode of manifesting itself.**

* Physical and moral diseases are cured in the same manner.   Why does the brilliant planet Jupiter disappear in the twilight from the eyes of him who gazes at it?   Because a similar but more potent power, the light of breaking day, then acts upon these organs.   With what are we in the habit of flattering the olfactory nerves when offended by disagreeable odours?   With snuff, which affects the nose in a similar manner, but more powerfully.   Neither music nor confectionary will overcome the disgust of smelling, because these objects have affinity with the nerves of other senses.   By what means does the soldier cunningly remove from the ears of the compassionate spectator the cries of him who runs the gauntlet?   By the piercing tones of the fife, coupled with the noise of the drum.   By what means do they drown the distant roar of the enemy's cannon, which carries terror to the heart of the soldier?   By the deep-mouthed clamour of the big drum.   Neither the compassion nor the terror could be suppressed by reprimands or a distribution of brilliant uniforms.   In the same manner, mourning and sadness are extinguished in the soul when the news reach us (even though they were false) of a still greater misfortune occurring to another.   The evils resulting from an excess of joy are mitigated by coffee, which, of itself, disposes the mind to impressions that are happy.   The Germans, a nation which had for centuries been plunged in apathy and slavery by their princes—it was not till after they had been bowed to the dust by the tyranny of the French invader, that a sentiment of the dignity of man could be awakened within them, or that they could once more arise from their abject condition.

The curative virtues of medicines depend solely upon the resemblance that their symptoms bear to those of the disease.

§ 27.   The curative powers of medicines are therefore grounded upon the faculty which they possess of creating symptoms similar to those of the disease itself, but which are of a more intense nature.   (§ 12—26.)   It necessarily follows, that disease cannot be destroyed or cured in a certain, radical, prompt and permanent manner, but by the aid of a medicine which is capable of exciting the entire group of symptoms which bear the closest resemblance to those of the disease, but which possess a still greater degree of energy.

Some explanation of this therapeutic law of nature.

§ 28. As this therapeutic law of nature clearly manifests itself in every accurate experiment and research, it consequently becomes an established fact, however unsatisfactory may be the scientific theory of the manner in which it takes place. I attach no value whatever to any explanation that could be given on this head; yet the following view of the subject appears to me to be the most reasonable, because it is founded upon experimental premises.

§ 29. *Every disease (which does not belong exclusively to surgery) being a purely dynamic and peculiar change of the vital powers in regard to the manner in which they accomplish sensation and action, a change that expresses itself by symptoms which are perceptible to the senses, it therefore follows, that the homœopathic medicinal agent, selected by a skilful physician, will convert it into another medicinal disease which is analogous, but rather more intense.* * *By this means, the natural morbific power which had previously existed, and which was nothing more than a dynamic power without substance, terminates, while the medicinal disease which usurps its place being of such a nature as to be easily subdued by the vital powers, is likewise extinguished in its turn, leaving in its primitive state of integrity and health the essence or substance which animates and preserves the body.* This hypothesis, which is highly probable, rests upon the following facts.

* The brief operation of the artificial morbific powers, which are denominated medicinal, although they are stronger than natural diseases, renders it possible that they may, nevertheless, be more easily overpowered by the vital energies than the latter, which are weaker. Natural diseases, simply because of their more tedious and burthensome operation, (as psora, syphilis, sycosis,) cannot be overcome or extinguished by the unaided vital energies, until these are more strongly aroused by the physician, through the medium of a very similar yet more powerful morbific agent (a homœopathic medicine). Such an agent, upon its administration, urges, as it were, the insensate, instinctive vital energies, and is substituted for the natural morbid affection hitherto existing. The vital energies now become affected by the medicine alone, yet transiently; because its effect (that is to say, the natural course of the medicinal disease thereby excited) is of short duration. Those chronic diseases

which (according to § 46) are destroyed on the appearance of small-pox and measles, (both of which run a course of a few weeks only,) furnish similar instances of cure.

The human body is much more prone to undergo derangement from the action of medicines than from that of natural disease.

§ 30. Medicines (particularly as it depends on us to vary the doses according to our own will) appear to have greater power in affecting the state of health than the natural morbific irritation; for natural diseases are cured and subdued by appropriate medicines.

§ 31. The physical and moral powers, which are called morbific agents, do not possess the faculty of changing the state of health unconditionally;* we do not fall sick beneath their influence before the economy is sufficiently disposed and laid open to the attack of morbific causes, and will allow itself to be placed by them in a state where the sensations which they undergo, and the actions which they perform, are different from those which belong to it in the normal state. These powers, therefore, do not excite disease in all men, nor are they at all times the cause of it in the same individual..

* When I say that disease is an aberration or a discord in the state of health, I do not pretend by that to give a metaphysical explanation of the immediate essence of diseases generally, or of any morbid case in particular. In making use of this term, I merely intend to point at that which diseases are not, and cannot be; or to express what I have just proved, that they are not mechanical or chemical changes of the material substance of the body, that they do not depend upon a morbific material principle, and that they are solely spiritual and dynamic changes of the animal economy.

§ 32. But it is quite otherwise with the artificial morbific powers which we call medicines. Every real medicine will at *all* times, and under *every* circumstance, work upon *every* living individual, and excite in him the symptoms that are peculiar to it, (so as to be clearly manifest to the senses when the dose is powerful enough,) to such a degree, that the whole of the system is always (*unconditionally*) attacked, and, in a manner, infected by the medicinal disease, which, as I have before said, is not at all the case in natural diseases.

§ 33. It is therefore fully proved by every experiment,* and observation, that the state of health is far more susceptible of

derangement from the effects of medicinal powers than from
the influence of morbific principles and contagious miasms;
or what is the same thing, the *ordinary morbific principles have
only a conditional and often very subordinate influence, while the
medicinal powers exercise one that is absolute, direct, and greatly
superior to that of the former.*

* The following is a striking observation of the kind directly in point:
previously to the year 1801, the genuine smooth scarlet fever of Sydenham
prevailed epidemically among children, and attacked all, without exception,
who had not escaped the disease in a former epidemic; whereas, every child who
was exposed to one of the kind which came under my observation in Königs-
lutter, remained exempt from this highly infectious disease, if it had timely
taken a very small dose of belladonna. When a medicine can thus evince a
prophylactic property against the infection of a prevalent disease, it must
exercise a predominating influence over the vital power.

*The truth of the homœopathic law is shown by the inefficacy of non-homœo-
pathic treatment in the cure of diseases that are of long standing, and
likewise by the fact that either of two natural dissimilar diseases co-exist-
ing in the body, cannot annihilate or cure the other.*

§ 34. In artificial diseases produced by medicines, it is not
the greater degree of intensity that imparts to them the power
they possess of curing those which are natural. In order that
the cure may be effected, it is indispensable that the medicines be able to produce in the human body an *artificial disease, similar* to that which is to be cured; for it is this resemblance alone, joined to the greater degree of intensity of the
artificial disease, that gives to the latter the faculty of substituting itself in the place of the former, and thus obliterating it.
This is so far a fact, that even nature herself cannot cure an
existing disease by the excitement of a new one that is dissimilar, be the intensity of the latter ever so great; in the same
manner the physician is incapable of effecting a cure when
he applies medicines that have not the power of creating in
healthy persons a morbid state, *resembling the disease* which is
before him.

§ 35. In order to illustrate these facts, we will examine
successively in three different cases the proceedings of nature
where two natural diseases that are dissimilar meet together
in the same patient, and also the results of the ordinary treatment of disease with allœopathic medicines which are inca-

pable of exciting an artificial morbid state, similar to that of
the disease which is to be cured. This examination will fully
prove, on the one hand, that it is not even in the power of nature herself to cure an existing disease by one that is dissimilar, be the intensity of the latter ever so great ; and on the
other, that even the most energetic medicines, when not
homœopathic, are incapable of effecting a cure.

*I. A disease, existing in the human body, prevents the accession of a new and
dissimilar one, if the former be of equal intensity to, or greater, than the
latter.*

§ 36. I. If the two *dissimilar* diseases which meet together
in the human body have an unequal power, or if the *oldest* of
them is *stronger* than the other, the new disease will be repulsed from the body by that which existed before it, and will
not be able to establish itself there. Thus a person already
afflicted with a severe chronic disease, will never be subject
to an attack of slight autumnal dysentery or any other epidemic. According to Larry,* the plague peculiar to the
Levant never breaks out in places where scurvy prevails, nor
does it ever infect those who labour under herpetic diseases.
According to Jenner, the rickets prevent vaccination from
taking effect, and Hildebrand informs us that persons suffering under phthisis are never attacked with epidemic fevers,
except when the latter are extremely violent.

* Mem. and Observ. in the Description of Egypt, tom. i.

*Thus, non-homœopathic treatment, which is not violent, leaves the chronic
disease unaltered.*

§ 37. In the same manner, a chronic disease, of long standing, will not yield to the *ordinary mode of cure* by *alœopathic*
remedies, that is to say, by medicines which are incapable of
producing in healthy persons a state analogous to that by
which it is characterized. It resists a treatment of this kind,
provided it be not too violent, even prolonged during several
years. Practice verifies this assertion, it therefore requires
no examples to support it.

*II. Or, a new and more intense disease suspends a prior and dissimilar one,
already existing in the body, only so long as the former continues, but it
never cures it.*

§ 38. II. If the *new* disease, which is *dissimilar* to the old, be *more powerful* than the latter, it will then cause its suspension until the new disease has either performed its own course or is cured ; but then the old disease *re-appears.* We are informed by Tulpius,[1] that two children having contracted tinea, ceased to experience any further attacks of epilepsy to which they had till then been subject ; but as soon as the eruption of the head was removed, they were again attacked as before. Schœpf saw the itch disappear when scurvy manifested itself, and return again after the cure of the latter disease.[2] A violent typhus has suspended the progress of ulcerous phthisis, which resumed its march immediately after the cessation of the typhoid disease.[3] When madness manifests itself during a pulmonary disease, it effaces the phthisis with all its symptoms ; but when the mental alienation ceases, the pulmonary disease again rears its head and kills the patient.[4] Where the measles and the small-pox exist together, and have both attacked the same infant, it is usual for the measles, which have already declared themselves, to be arrested by the small-pox which bursts forth, and not to resume their course until after the cure of the latter ; on the other hand, Manget[5] has also seen the small-pox, which had fully developed itself after inoculation, suspended during four days by the measles which intervened, and after the desquamation of which, it revived again to run its course. The eruption of measles on the sixth day after inoculation has been known to arrest the inflammatory operation of the latter, and the small-pox did not break out until the other exanthema had accomplished its seven days' course.[6] In an epidemic, the measles broke out among several patients four or five days after inoculation, and retarded until their entire disappearance the eruption of the small-pox, which subsequently proceeded in a regular manner.[7] The true scarlet fever of Sydenham,[8] with angina, was arrested on the fourth day by the manifestation of the cow-pock, which went through its natural course ; and not before its termination did the scarlet fever manifest itself again. But as these two diseases appear to be of equal force, the cow-pock has likewise been seen to suspend itself on the eighth day by the eruption of genuine scarlatina, and the red areola was effaced until the scarlatina had terminated its career, at which moment the cow-pock resumed its course, and terminated regu-

larly.[9] The cow-pock was on the point of attaining to its
state of perfection on the eighth day, when measles broke out,
which immediately rendered it stationary, and not before the
desquamation of which did it resume and finish its course; so
that, according to the report of Kortum,[10] it presented on the
sixteenth day the aspect which it usually wears on the tenth.
The vaccine virus has been known to infect the system even
where the measles had already made their appearance, but it
did not pursue its course until the measles had passed away;
for this we have also the authority of Kortum.[11]

I have myself had an opportunity of seeing a parotid angina
disappear immediately after the development of the cow-pock.
It was not till after the cow-pock had terminated, and the disappearance of the red areola of the vesicles, that a great
swelling, attended with fever, manifested itself in the parotid
and sub-maxillary glands, which ran its ordinary course of
seven days.

*It is the same in all diseases that are dissimilar; the stronger
one suspends the weaker,* (except in cases where they blend
together, which rarely occurs in acute diseases); *but they
never cure each other reciprocally.*

[1] Obs. lib. i. obs. 8.   [2] In Hufeland's Journal, XV. ii.
[3] Chevalier, in Hufeland's neuesten Annalen der franz. Heilkunde. ii. p. 192.
[4] Mania phthisi superveniens eam cum omnibus suis phænomenis aufert,
verum mox redit phthisis et occidit, abeunte mania. Reil, Memorabilia Fasc.
III. v. p. 171.
[5] Edinb. Med. Comment. T. I. i.
[6] J. Hunter on the Venereal Disease.
[7] Rainey, Edinb. Med. Comment. iii, p. 480.
[8] It has also been very accurately described by Withering and Plenciz, and
differs greatly from purpura, to which they often give the name of scarlet
fever Only within the last few years have both, originally very different
diseases, approached more or less to each other in their symptoms.
[9] Jenner, in the Annals of Medicine for August, 1800, p. 747.
[10] In Hufeland's Journal, XX. iii. p. 50.   [11] Loc. cit.

*In the same manner, violent treatment with allœopathic remedies never cures
a chronic disease, but merely suspends it during the continuance of the
powerful action of a medicine incapable of exciting symptoms similar to
those of the disease; but afterwards, the latter re-appears even more intense
than before.*

§ 39. The ordinary schools of medicine have witnessed all
these effects during whole centuries. They have seen that

nature was never in any instance capable of curing a disease
by adding another, whatever degree of intensity the latter
might possess, if it was *not similar* to the pre-existing disease.
What opinion, then, ought we to form of these schools of
medicine, which continued, notwithstanding, to treat chronic
diseases with allœopathic remedies—that is to say, with substances which were scarcely ever able to excite anything else
but a disease *dissimilar* to the affection that was to be cured?
And though physicians had never before regarded nature with
a due share of attention, would it not still have been possible
for them to discover, from the miserable results of their mode
of treatment, that they were pursuing a wrong path, which
could only lead them still farther from their purpose? Could
they not see that in having recourse (according to their usual
practice) to violent allœopathic remedies in chronic diseases,
they did nothing more than provoke an artificial malady *dissimilar* to the primitive disease, which certainly had the effect
of extinguishing the latter so long as the other continued to
exist, but which suffered it to re-appear as soon as the diminished powers of the patient could no longer support the vigorous attacks of allœopathy on the vital principle? It is in this
manner that strong purgatives, frequently repeated, cause
eruptions of the skin to disappear pretty quickly; but when
the patient can no longer endure the dissimilar disease that
has been violently kindled in the vitals, and is compelled to
discontinue the purgatives, then the cutaneous eruption either
flourishes again in its former vigour, or the internal psoric
affection manifests itself by some bad symptom or another,
while, in addition to the primitive malady, (which is not in the
least degree diminished,) indigestion ensues, and the vital
powers are exhausted. Thus, also, when ordinary physicians
insert setons, and excite ulceration of the surface of the body,
for the purpose of destroying chronic diseases, they *never*
accomplish the object they have in view—that is to say, they
never perform a cure, because those factitious cutaneous ulcers
are perfectly foreign and allœopathic to the internal disease;
but the irritation produced by many cauteries being often a
more powerful disease than the primitive morbid state,
(although at the same time dissimilar,) it frequently has the
power of silencing the latter for a short time, which is nothing

more than a *suspension* of the disease obtained at the expense
of the patient, whose powers are thereby gradually diminished.
An epilepsy which had been suppressed during several years
by issues, constantly re-appeared more violent than before
whenever the exuditories were allowed to heal up, as attested
by Pechlin* and others. But purgatives are no more allœopathic in regard to psora, or issues in respect of epilepsy, than
the compounds of unknown ingredients employed till the present time in ordinary practice are so in relation to the other
innumerable forms of disease. These mixtures do nothing
more than weaken the patient, and suspend the evil for a very
short space of time without being able to cure it, while their
continued and repeated use, as it frequently happens, adds a
new disease to the old one.

* Obs. Phys. Med. lib. 2, obs. 30.

*III. Or, the new disease, after having acted for a considerable time on the sys-
tem, joins itself finally to the old one, which is dissimilar, and thence results
a complication of two different maladies, either of which is incapable of annihilating or curing the other.*

§ 40. III. Or it sometimes occurs that the *new disease*, after
having acted for a considerable period upon the system, joins
itself finally to the old dissimilar one, presenting together a
complicated form of disease, but in such a manner that each
of them, notwithstanding, occupies a particular region of the
economy, installing itself in those organs with which it sym-
pathises, and abandoning the others to the diseases that are
dissimilar. Thus a venereal affection may turn to one that is
psoric, and *vice versa*. *These two diseases being dissimilar, they
are incapable of annihilating or curing each other.* Venereal
symptoms are effaced and suspended, in the first instance, as
soon as a psoric eruption commences ; but, in the progress of
time, the venereal affection being at least quite as powerful
as the psoric, the two unite together[1]—that is to say, each
seizes merely upon those parts of the organism that are appropriate to it individually, by which the patient is rendered
worse, and the cure more difficult than before. In a case
where two contagious acute diseases meet together, bearing
no analogy to each other, (such as, for example, the small-
pox and the measles,) one of them ordinarily suspends the
other, as before stated. However, there have been some ex-

traordinary instances in violent epidemic diseases, where two dissimilar acute maladies have simultaneously attacked the body of the same individual, and become, so to express it, complicated for a short time. In an epidemic where the small-pox and the measles reigned together, there were about three hundred cases in which one of these maladies suspended the other, and in which the measles did not break forth until twenty days after the eruption of the small-pox, and the latter till from seventeen to eighteen days after that of the measles—that is to say, until after the first disease had run its entire course; but there was a single instance in which P. Russell[2] met with these two dissimilar maladies simultaneously in the same patient. / Rainey[3] saw the small-pox and the measles together in two little girls; and J. Maurice[4] remarks that he never met with more than two instances of this kind in the whole course of his practice. Similar examples may be found in Ettmüller,[5] and a few other writers. Zencker[6] saw the cow-pock pursue its course in a regular manner conjointly with measles and purpura: and Jenner likewise observed it pursue its course tranquilly in the midst of a mercurial treatment directed against the venereal disease.

[1] The cures which I performed of these kinds of complicated diseases, together with the accurate experiments which I have made, have convinced me that they do not arise from an amalgamation of two diseases; but that the latter exist *separately* in the organism, each occupying the parts that are most in harmony with it. In short, the cure is effected in a very complete manner by administering alternately, and at the proper time, mercurials, and antipsorics, each according to its appropriate dose and preparation.

[2] Transactions of a Society for the Improvement of Med. and Chir. Knowledge, vol. ii.

[3] Med. Comment. of Edinb. iii. p. 480.

[4] Med. and Phys. Journal, 1805.

[5] Opera, ii. p. i. cap. 10.

[6] In Hufeland's Journal, xvii.

Much more frequently than a superadded natural disease, an artificial one, which is occasioned by the long continued use of violent and unsuitable allæopathic remedies, is combined with the dissimilar prior and natural disease (the dissimilarity consequently rendering it incurable by means of the artificial malady,) and the patient becomes doubly diseased.

§ 41. The complication or co-existence of several diseases in the same patient, resulting from a long use of medicines that were not homœopathic, is far more frequent than those to which nature herself has given birth. The continued application of inappropriate medicines finishes by adding to the natural disease which it is intended to cure, such fresh morbid symptoms as those remedies are capable of exciting according to the nature of their special properties. These symptoms not being capable of curing by analogous counter irritation, (that is to say, homœopathically,) a chronic disease to which they bear no similitude, gradually associate themselves to the latter, and thus add a new factitious disease to the old one, so that the patient becomes considerably worse and far more difficult to cure. There are many observations and cases cited in the medical journals and treatises that support this assertion. One proof of it is also to be met with in the frequent cases of the venereal chancrous disease, especially when complicated with psora, and even with gonorrhea, sycotica, which, far from being cured by considerable and repeated doses of inappropriate mercurial preparations, station themselves in the organism alongside of the chronic mercurial disease which develops itself gradually,* and form together a monstrous complication generally designated by the name of masked syphilis, (pseudo-syphilis,) a state of disease which if not absolutely incurable, cannot at least but with the greatest difficulty be changed to that of health.

* For besides the morbid symptoms analogous to those of the venereal disease, which would be capable of curing the same homœopathically, mercury produces a crowd of others which bear no resemblance whatever to those of syphilis, and which, when administered in large doses, especially where there is a complication with psora, as is frequently the case, engenders fresh evils, and commits terrible ravages on the body.

The diseases thus complicated by reason of their dissimilarity, assume different places in the organism to which they are severally adapted.

§ 42. Nature, as I have before said, sometimes permits the coincidence of two and even three spontaneous diseases in one and the same body ; but it must be observed, that this complication never takes place but in diseases that are dissimilar, and which, according to the eternal laws of nature, cannot annihilate or cure each other reciprocally. Apparently this is executed in such a manner that the two or three diseases divide, if we may so express it, the organism between them, and each takes possession of the parts that are best suited to it individually; a division which, in consequence of the want of similitude between them, can very well take place without doing injury to the unity of the vital principle.

But very different is the result, where a new disease that is similar and stronger is superadded to the old one, for in that case the former annihilates and cures the latter.

§ 43. But the result is very different when two diseases that are similar meet together in the organism—that is to say, when an analogous but more powerful disease joins itself to the pre-existing malady. It is true that we here see how a cure is performed according to nature, and how man is to proceed in effecting the same object.

§ 44. Two diseases that *resemble* each other closely can neither *repel*, (as in the first of the three preceding hypotheses, I.,) nor *suspend* each other, (as in the second, II.,) so that the old one re-appears after the cessation of the new one: nor, finally, (as in the third, III.,) can they *exist beside each other* in the same organism, and form a *double* or complicated disease.

This phenomenon explained.

§ 45. No ! Two diseases that differ greatly in their species,[1] but which bear a strong resemblance in their development and effects—that is to say, in the symptoms which they produce, always mutually destroy each other when they meet together in the system. The stronger annihilates the weaker ; nor is it difficult to conceive how this is performed. Two dissimilar diseases may co-exist in the body, because their dissimilitude would allow of their occupying two distinct regions. But, in the present case, the stronger disease which makes its appearance, exercises an influence upon the *same* parts as the old one, and even throws itself, in preference, upon those which have till now been attacked by the latter; so that the old disease, finding no other organ to act upon, is necessarily extinguished.[2] Or, to express it in other terms, as soon as the vital powers, which have till then been deranged by a morbific cause, are attacked with greater energy by a

new power very analogous to the former, but more intense,
they no longer receive any impression but from the latter,
while the preceding one, reduced to a state of mere dynamic
power without matter, must cease to exist.

[1] See the note attached to § 26.
[2] In the same way that the light of a lamp is rapidly effaced from the retina
by a sunbeam which strikes the eye with greater force.

*Examples of the cure of chronic diseases, by the accidental accession of
another disease, similar and more intense.*

§ 46. Many examples might be adduced where nature has
cured diseases homœopathically by other diseases which excited similar symptoms. But if precise and indisputable facts
alone be required, it will be necessary to confine ourselves to
the few diseases which arise from some permanent miasm,
and constantly preserve their identity, for which reason they
ought to receive a distinct appellation.

The foremost that presents itself among these affections is
the small-pox, so famous for the violence and number of its
symptoms, and which has cured a multitude of diseases that
were characterized by symptoms similar to its own.

Violent ophthalmia, extending even to the loss of sight, is
one of the most ordinary occurrences in the small-pox;
whereas Dezoteux[1] and Leroy[2] have each reported cases of
chronic ophthalmia which were cured in a perfect and permanent manner by inoculation.

A case of blindness of two years' standing brought on by
the metastasis of tinea, was, according to Klein,[3] perfectly
cured by the small-pox. How often has the small-pox cured
deafness and oppressed respiration? J. F. Closs[4] has seen it
cure both these affections when it had reached its highest
state of intensity.

Considerable enlargement of the testicle is a frequent symptom in small-pox, and, according to Klein,[5] it has been known
to cure homœopathically a large hard swelling of the left
testicle, the consequence of a contusion. Another observer[6]
has seen it cure a similar swelling of the testicle.

Dysentery is one of the bad symptoms which occur in small-
pox—for this reason it cures the former disease homœopathically, as in a case reported by F. Wendt.[7]

The small-pox, which comes on after vaccination, destroys the latter immediately, and does not permit it to arrive at perfection, both because it is more powerful than the cow-pock, and bears a close resemblance to it. By the same reason, when the cow-pock approaches to its term of maturity, it diminishes and softens, in a very great degree, the small-pox which has just broken out, and causes it to assume a milder form, as witnessed by Mühry[8] and many others.

The cow-pock, in addition to the vesicles which protect from small-pox, excites also a general cutaneous eruption of another kind. This exanthema consists of sharp-pointed pimples, usually small, seldom large and suppurating, dry, resting upon a small red areola, frequently interspersed with small round spots of a red colour, and sometimes attended with severe itching. In many children it precedes by several days the appearance of the red areola of the cow-pock. But most often it manifests itself afterwards, and disappears in a few days, leaving small hard red spots on the skin. It is by reason of this other exanthema, and the analogy which it bears to the same, that the cow-pock, the moment it takes, removes in a permanent manner those cutaneous eruptions which exist in some children, and which are often troublesome and of long standing. This has been attested by numerous observers.[9]

Vaccination, whose special symptom is a swelling of the arm,[10] cured, after its eruption, the *tumefaction* of an arm that was half paralyzed.[11]

The vaccine fever, which takes place at the period of the formation of the red areola, has, according to the information of Hardège,[12] cured two cases of intermittent fever homœopathically; which confirms the remark formerly made by J. Hunter,[13] that two fevers (or diseases that are similar) can never exist together in the body.†

The measles and hooping cough resemble each other both in regard to the fever and the character of the cough. This was the reason that Bosquillon[14] observed, during an epidemic of measles and hooping-cough, that among the children who had the former there were many entirely free from the latter. All of them would have been exempt from hooping-cough for ever after, and also beyond the reach of the contagion of measles, if the hooping-cough was not a disease that only re-

sembled the measles partially—that is, if it produced an eruption of the skin analogous to that of the latter; thus the
measles are able to preserve but a certain number of children
homœopathically from the hooping-cough, nor can they do this
for a longer period than during the continuance of the reigning epidemic.

But when the measles come in contact with a disease that
resembles them in the principal symptom, viz. the eruption,
they can beyond a doubt annihilate and cure it homœopathically. It was under such circumstances that the eruption of
measles cured a chronic tetter[15] in a prompt, durable, and
perfect manner, as observed by Kortum.[16] A miliary eruption
that covered the neck, face, and arms, during a period of six
years, attended with insupportable heat, and which returned
at every change of weather, was reduced to a simple swelling
of the skin on the appearance of measles; after the cessation
of the latter, the miliary eruption was cured and never re-
appeared.[17]

[1] Traité de l'Inoculation, p. 189.
[2] Heilkunde für Mütter, (Medical Treatise for the use of Mothers,) p. 384.
[3] Interpres Clinicus, p 293.
[4] Neue Heilart der Kinderpocken, (New System for the Cure of Small-
pox,) Ulm, 1769, p. 68, and Specim. Obs. No. 18.
[5] Loc. cit.
[6] Nov. Act. Nat. Cur. vol. i. obs. 22.
[7] Nachricht von dem Krankeninstitut (Directions of the Medical Board)
at Erlangen, 1783.
[8] In R. Willan on Vaccination.
[9] Particularly Clavier, Hurel, and Desormeaux, in the Bulletin des Sc.
Med. de l'Eure, 1808. Journal de Médecine continué, xv. 206.
[10] Balhorn, in Hufeland's Journal, X. ii.
[11] Stevenson, in Duncan, Annals of Med. Mustr. ii. vol. i. sect. 2. No. 9.
[12] In Hufeland's Journal, xxiii.
[13] Ueber die venerische Krankheit, (on the Venereal Disease,) p. 4.
† In the former editions of the Organon, I have cited cases where chronic
diseases have been cured by psora, which, according to the discoveries I have
made known in the first part of my *Treatise on Chronic Diseases*, can only
be partially regarded as homœopathic cures. The great affections which
were thus obliterated, (such as suffocating asthma and phthisis of many years'
standing,) already owed their origin to some psoric cause. The symptoms of
a psoric eruption of long standing, which were completely developed in the
system, and threatened the life of the patient, were reduced by the appearance of a psoric eruption caused by a new infection, to the simple form of

primitive psora, by which means the old disease, with its alarming symptoms, were removed. This return to the primitive form cannot, therefore, be regarded as a homœopathic cure of the old psora but in this sense, that the new infection places the patient in a much more favourable way of being subsequently cured of the entire psora by antipsoric medicines.

¹⁴ Cullen's Elements of Pract. Med. part ii. l. 3, ch. 7.
¹⁵ Or at least this symptom was removed.
¹⁶ In Hufeland's Journal, XX. ii. p. 50.
¹⁷ Rau, loc. cit. p. 85.

Of any two diseases, which occur in the ordinary course of nature, it is only that one whose symptoms are similar to the other, which can cure or destroy it. This faculty never belongs to a dissimilar disease. Hence the physician may learn what are the remedies with which he can effect a certain cure, that is to say, with none but such as are homœopathic.

§ 47. No instructions can be more simple and persuasive than these, to direct the physician in the choice of the substances (medicines) which are capable of exciting artificial diseases, in order that he may be enabled to cure in a prompt and durable manner according to the course of nature.

§ 48. All the preceding examples prove to us that neither the efforts of nature, nor the skill of the physician, have ever been able to cure a disease by a dissimilar morbific power, whatever energy the latter may have possessed ; also, that a cure is not to be obtained but by a morbific power capable of producing *symptoms that are similar, and, at the same time, a little stronger.* The cause of this rests with the eternal and irrevocable law of nature, which was hitherto not understood.

§ 49. We should have met with a much greater number of those truly natural homœopathic cures, if, on the one hand, observers had been more attentive to the subject, and, on the other, nature had at her disposal more diseases capable of effecting homœopathic cures.

Nature affords but few instances in which one disease can homœopathically destroy another, and her remedial resources in this way are encumbered by many inconveniences.

§ 50. Even nature herself has no other homœopathic agents at her command than the miasmatic diseases which always retain their identity, such as itch, measles, and small-pox.* But of these morbific powers, the small-pox and the

9

measles are more dangerous and terrific than the maladies which they cure ; and the other, psora, demands itself, after the performance of a cure, the application of a remedy that is capable of annihilating it in its turn : both of these are circumstances that render their use as homœopathic remedies difficult, uncertain, and dangerous. And how few are the diseases to which man is subject, that would find their homœopathic cure in psora, measles, or small-pox ! Nature can, therefore, cure but a very limited number of diseases with those hazardous remedies. Their use is attended with considerable danger to the patient, because the doses of these morbific agents cannot be varied according to circumstances, as in the case with doses of medicine ; and in curing an analogous disease of long standing, they weigh down the patient with the dangerous burden of psora, measles, and small-pox. Notwithstanding this, we have many examples where their favourable junction has produced the most perfect homœopathic cures, which are a living commentary upon the sole therapeutic law of nature—*cure with medicines that are capable of exciting symptoms analogous to those of the disease itself.*

* And the exanthematic miasm which is contained in the cow-pock lymph.

On the other hand, the physician is possessed of innumerable curative agents, greatly preferable to those.

§ 51. These facts will more than suffice to reveal to the understandings of men the great law which has just been declared. And behold the advantage which man has here over rude nature, whose acts are not guided by reflection ! How are the homœopathic morbific powers multiplied in the various medicines which are spread over the creation, all of which are at his disposal, and may be brought to the relief of his suffering fellow-mortals ! With these, he can create morbid symptoms as varied as the countless natural diseases which they are to cure. With such precious resources at his command, there can be no necessity for those violent attacks upon the organism to extirpate an old and obstinate disease ; and the transition from the state of suffering to that of durable health is effected in a gentle, imperceptible, and often speedy manner.

From the process employed by nature, to which we have just adverted, the physician may deduce the doctrine of curing diseases by no other remedies than such as are homœopathic, and not with those of another kind, (allœopathic,) which never cure, but only injure the patient.

§ 52. After such evidence and examples, it is impossible for any reasonable physician to persevere in the ordinary allœopathic treatment, or continue to apply remedies whose effects have no direct or homœopathic relation with the chronic disease that is to be cured, and which attack the body in the parts that are least diseased, by exciting evacuations, counter-irritation, derivations, &c.* It is impossible that he can persist in the adoption of a method which consists in exciting, at the expense of the powers of the patient, the appearance of a morbid state entirely different from the primitive affection, by administering strong doses of mixtures which are of the most part composed of drugs whose effects are unknown. The use of such mixtures can have no other result but that which proceeds from the general law of nature when one dissimilar disease joins itself to another in the animal economy—that is to say, *the chronic affection, far from being cured, is, on the contrary, always aggravated.* Three different effects may then take place :—1st. If the allœopathic treatment, though of long duration, be gentle, the natural disease remains unchanged, and the patient will only have lost a portion of his strength, because, as we have seen before, the disease which already exists in the body will not permit a new *dissimilar* one that is weaker to establish itself there likewise. 2d. When the economy is attacked with violence by allœopathic medicines, the primitive disease will yield for a time ; but it re-appears, with at least the same degree of vigour as before, the moment this treatment is interrupted, because, as before stated, of two concurrent diseases, the new one, which is the stronger, destroys and suspends for a time that which existed before it, which is weaker and *dissimilar.* 3d. Finally, if large doses of allœopathic medicines be continued for a length of time, this treatment only adds a new factitious disease without ever curing the primitive one, and renders the cure still more difficult ; because, as we have already seen, when two dissimilar chronic affections of equal intensity meet together, one takes up its station beside the other in the system, and both are simultaneously established.

* See the introduction, "A View," etc., and my book—Die Allœopathie, ein Wort der Warnung an Kranke jeder Art.—Leipzig, bei Baumgärtner.

There are only three possible methods of employing medicines in diseases, viz.

§ 53. These cures are, as we see, performed solely by means of homœopathy, which we have at length attained to, by consulting reason and taking experience for our guide (§ 7—25). By this method alone can we cure disease in the most speedy, certain, and permanent manner, because it is grounded upon an eternal and unerring law of nature.

I. The homœopathic, which only is salutary and efficacious.

§ 54. I have before remarked (§ 43—49) that there is no true method but the *homœopathic;* because, of the only three modes of employing medicines in disease, this alone leads in a direct line to a mild, safe, and durable cure, without either injuring the patient or diminishing his strength.

II. The allœopathic or heteropathic.

§ 55. The second mode of employing medicines in disease, is that which I term the *allœopathic,* or *heteropathic,* which has been in general use till the present time. Without ever regarding that which is really diseased in the body, it attacks those parts which are sound, in order to draw off the malady from another quarter, and direct it towards the latter. I have already treated of this method in the Introduction, and therefore will not speak of it farther.

III. The antipathic or enantiopathic, which is merely palliative.

§ 56. The third and last mode of employing medicines in disease is the *antipathic, enantiopathic,* or *palliative.* By this method, physicians have, till the present time, succeeded in affording *apparent* relief, and gained the confidence of their patients by deluding them with a temporary suspension of their sufferings. We will now show its inefficacy, and to what extent it is even injurious in diseases that run their course rapidly. In fact, this is the only feature, in the treatment employed by allœopathists, that has any direct reference to the sufferings occasioned by the natural disease. But in what does this reference consist? In precisely that which ought most to be avoided if we would not delude and mock the patient.

An exposition of the method of cure where a remedy producing a contrary ef-fect (contraria contrariis) is prescribed against a single symptom of the disease.—Examples.

§ 57. An ordinary physician who proceeds upon the antipathic method, pays attention to one symptom only—that of which the patient complains loudest, and neglects all the others, however numerous. He prescribes against this symptom a medicine that is known to produce the very opposite effect; for, according to the axiom *contraria contrariis*, laid down fifteen hundred years ago by the old schools of medicine, it is from this remedy that he expects the most speedy relief (palliative.) Accordingly, he administers strong doses of opium in pains of every description, because this substance rapidly benumbs the feeling. He prescribes the same drug in diarrhœa, because in a short time it stops the peristaltic movement of the intestinal canal, and renders it insensible. He administers it likewise in cases of insomnolence, because it produces a state of hebetude and stupor. He employs purgatives when the patient has for a long time been tormented with constipation. He plunges a hand that has received a burn into cold water, because its icy quality appears suddenly to remove the pain as if by enchantment. When a patient complains of a sense of cold and loss of vital heat, he places him in a warm bath, whereby heat is immediately restored. Any one complaining of habitual weakness, is advised to take wine, which immediately re-animates and appears to refresh him. Some other antipathics—that is to say, medicines opposed to the symptoms—are likewise employed; but independent of those I have just enumerated, there are not many, because ordinary physicians are only acquainted with the peculiar and primitive effects of a very small number of medicines.

This antipathic method is not merely defective because it is directed against an individual symptom only, but also, because in chronic diseases, after having apparently diminished the evil for a time, this temporary abatement is followed by a real aggravation of the symptoms.

§ 58. I will pass over the defect (see the note to § 7) which

this method has in attaching itself to *but one of the symptoms,*
and consequently but to a small part of the whole, a circumstance from which nothing could evidently be expected for the
amelioration of the entire disease, which is the only thing the
patient aspires to.   I will now ask, if experience can show me
a single case where the application of these antipathic remedies in chronic or permanent diseases, and the short relief
which they have procured, has not been followed by a manifest aggravation, not only of the symptoms thus palliated in
the first instance, but what is more, of the entire disease?
Every one who has paid attention to the subject will concur
in saying, that after this slight antipathic amendment, which
lasts only for a short time, the condition of the patient *invariably becomes worse,* although the ordinary physician endeavours
to account for this too palpable augmentation, by attributing
it to the malignity of the primitive disease, which, according
to his account, only then began to manifest itself.*

* However unaccustomed physicians may have been till the present time
to make correct observations, it could not have escaped their notice, that disease infallibly increases after the use of palliatives. A striking example of
this nature is found in J. H. Schulze, (*Diss. qua corporis humani momenta-
nearum alterationum specimina quædam expenduntur. Halle,* 1741, § 28).
Something similar to this is attested by Willis (*Pharm. rat. sec.* 7. cap. i. p.
298) : *Opiata dolores atrocissimos plerumque sedant atque indolentiam......
procurant, eamque....aliquamdiu et pro stato quodam tempore continuant,
quo spatio elapso, dolores mox recrudescunt et brevi ad solitam ferociam au-
gentur.* And p. 295 :—*Exactis opii viribus illico redeunt tormina, nec atroci-
tatem suam remittunt, nisi dum ab eodem pharmaco rursus incantantur.*
J. Hunter (in his Treatise on the Venereal Disease, p. 13) says that
wine increases the energy of persons who are weak, without bestowing on
them any real vigour ; and that the vital powers sink afterwards in the same
proportion as they have been stimulated, so that the patient gains nothing by
it, but, on the contrary, loses the greater part of his strength.

Injurious consequences of some antipathic cures.

§ 59.   No severe symptom of a permanent disease has ever
been treated by these opposite remedies and palliatives, where
the evil did not re-appear after a few hours, more aggravated
than before.   Thus, to cure an habitual tendency to sleep
during the day, coffee was administered, the first effects of
which are excitement and insomnolence ; but the moment
that its first action was exhausted, the propensity to sleep

returned stronger than ever. When a person was subject to frequent waking at night, without any regard being paid to the other symptoms of the disease, opium was administered at bed-time, which, by virtue of its primitive action, produces sleep, stupor, and hebetude; but on the following night the evil only became still more aggravated in consequence. Alike regardless of the other symptoms, opium was administered in chronic diarrhœa, because its primitive effect is to constipate the bowels; but the alvine flux, after having been suspended for some time, re-appeared more grievous than before. Acute and frequent pains of all descriptions were momentarily calmed beneath the influence of opium, which blunts and benumbs the feeling; but they never failed to return with greater violence than before, or they were even sometimes replaced by another disease of a worse description. The ordinary physician knows no better remedy for a cough of long standing, which becomes worse at night, than opium, whose first effects remove all kinds of irritation; for the first night it may very well happen that the patient experiences some relief, but on the succeeding nights the cough returns more distressing than ever; and if the physician persists in combating it with the same palliative by gradually increasing the dose, nocturnal perspirations and fever will then be added to the previous complaint. It has been imagined, that tincture of cantharides, which stimulates the urinary passages, would remedy a weakness of the bladder, and the retention of urine which results from it; it may, indeed, effect some forced emissions of urine, but in the end the bladder is only rendered less irritable and less susceptible of contraction, while paralysis of the bladder is likely to follow. Physicians have flattered themselves that they could subdue an inveterate tendency to constipation by purgatives administered in large doses, which provoke frequent and abundant alvine evacuations; but the secondary effect of this treatment is generally that of constipating the bowels in a still greater degree. An ordinary physician prescribes wine as a remedy in chronic debility; but it is only the primitive action of this agent that is stimulating, and its definitive results are those of reducing the powers still more.

It has been imagined that bitters and spices would warm and strengthen the cold and inactive stomach; but the se-

condary effect of these heating palliatives is to increase the
inactivity of the gastric viscera. Warm baths have been
prescribed in cases of rigours and an habitual deficiency of the
vital heat ; but on coming out of the water, the patients are
still weaker, more incapable of receiving warmth, and more
subject to rigours than they were before. Immersion in cold
water instantly relieves the pain occasioned by a severe burn ;
subsequently, however, this pain is increased to an insupportable degree, and the inflammation extends to the neighbouring parts.* To cure gravedo of long standing, sternuta-
tories are prescribed, which excite the pituitary secretion ;
and it has not been perceived that the final result of this
method was always that of aggravating the evil which it was
intended to cure. Electricity and galvanism, which at first
exercise great influence upon the muscular system, quickly
restore activity to members that have for a long time been
feeble and nearly paralyzed : but the secondary effect is absolute annihilation of all muscular irritability, and entire paralysis. It has been said that venesection is a fit remedy to
stop long-continued congestions of blood in the head ; but this
mode is always succeeded by a still greater determination of
blood to the upper parts of the body. The sole remedy that
physicians in ordinary know to apply in cases where the
moral and physical powers are inactive and half paralyzed,
which are predominant symptoms in different kinds of typhus,
is valerian, administered in strong doses, because this plant
is one of the most powerful excitants they are acquainted
with ; but it escaped their notice, that the excitement which
valerian produces is merely its primitive effect, and after the
re-action of the organism, the stupor and the incapability of
motion—that is to say, the paralysis of the body, and the debility of the mind, increase—they have not observed that the
patients on whom they lavished doses of the antipathic valerian, are precisely those who have suffered the greatest mor-
tality. In short, the former schools of medicine have never
calculated how often the secondary effects of antipathic medicines have tended to increase the malady, or even bring on
something that was still worse, of which experience has given
us examples that are enough to inspire the soul with terror.

* See the close of the Introduction.

Where a palliative is employed, the gradual increase of the dose never cures a chronic disease, but renders the state of the patient worse.

§ 60. When these grievous consequences (which naturally might have been expected from the use of antipathic remedies) begin to manifest themselves, the ordinary physician imagines that he will be delivered from his embarrassment if he administers a stronger dose each time that the evil grows worse. But from this also, there results nothing but momentary relief, while from the necessity in which he sees himself of constantly augmenting the dose of the palliative, it sometimes follows that a still severer malady declares itself—sometimes that life is endangered, and even that the patient falls a sacrifice. A disease of long-standing or of inveteracy has *never been cured* by such means.

Wherefore, physicians ought to have inferred the utility of an opposite, and the only beneficial method, namely, that of homœopathy.

§ 61. *If physicians had been capable of reflecting upon the sad results of the application of antipathic remedies, they would long ago have arrived at the great truth, that a path directly opposite would lead them to a method of treatment by which they might cure disease perfectly and permanently.* They would then have discovered, that if a medicinal effect, contrary to the symptoms of the malady, (antipathic treatment,) only procures momentary relief, at the expiration of which the evil constantly grows worse ; by the same rule the inverse method—that is to say, the *homœopathic application of medicines,* administered according to the analogy existing between the symptoms they excite and those of the disease itself, substituting, at the same time, for the enormous doses that were in use, the smallest that could possibly be applied—must necessarily bring about a perfect and permanent cure. But notwithstanding all these arguments—notwithstanding the positive fact, that no physician ever performed a permanent cure in chronic diseases but in proportion as the prescriptions included some predominant homœopathic medicine—notwithstanding another fact no less clear, that nature never accomplished a speedy and perfect cure but by means of a *similar* disease which she added to the old one (§ 46) ; notwithstanding all this, physicians have, during so many centuries, never arrived at a truth on which alone depended the safety of the patient.

The reason that the palliative method is so pernicious, and the homœopathic alone salutary.

§ 62. The source of all these pernicious results of palliative antipathic treatment, and the salutary effects proceeding from the reverse method, the homœopathic, will be sufficiently explained in the following observations, which are drawn from experience, and a number of facts that have hitherto escaped the notice ef every other physician, although they were immediately before the view, perfectly evident in their nature, and of the deepest importance to the medical art.

Is founded upon the difference which exists between the primary action of every medicine, and the re-action, or secondary effects, produced by the living organism (the vital power).

§ 63. Every agent that acts upon the human economy, every medicine produces more or less some notable change in the existing state of the vital powers, or creates a certain modification in the health of man for a period of shorter or longer duration : this change is called the *primitive effect.* Although this is the joint effect of both a medicinal and a vital power, it belongs, notwithstanding, more particularly to the former, whose action is exercised upon the body. But our vital powers tend always to oppose their energy to this influence or impression. The effect that results from this, and which belongs to our conservative vital powers and their automatic force, bears the name of *secondary effect,* or *re-action.*

Explanation of the primitive and secondary effects.

§ 64. So long as the primitive effects of artificial morbific agents (medicines) continue their influence upon a healthy body, the vital power appears to play merely a passive part, as if it were compelled to undergo the impression of the medicine that is acting upon it from without. But, subsequently, this also appears, in a manner, to rouse itself. Then, if there exists any state directly contrary to the primitive effect, (*a*) the vital power manifests a tendency to produce one (*b*) that is proportionate to its own energy, and the degree of influence exercised by the morbid or medicinal agent ; and if there exists no state in nature that is directly contrary to this primitive effect, the vital power then seeks to gain the ascendency by destroying the change that has been operated upon it from without, (by the action of the medicine,) for which it substitutes its own natural state (*re-action*).

Examples of both.

§ 65. Examples of (*a*) are before the eyes of every one. A hand that has been bathed in hot water has, at first, a much greater share of heat than the other that has not undergone the immersion (primitive effect); but shortly after it is withdrawn from the water, and well dried, it becomes cold again, and in the end much colder than that on the opposite side (secondary effect). The great degree of heat that accrues from violent exercise (primitive effect,) is followed by shivering and cold (secondary effect). A man who has overheated himself by drinking copiously of wine (primitive effect) finds, on the next day, even the slightest current of air too cold for him (secondary effect). An arm that has been immersed for any length of time in freezing water, is at first much paler and colder than the other (primitive effect) ; but let it be withdrawn from the water, and carefully dried, it will not only become warmer than the other, but even burning hot, red, and inflamed (secondary effect). Strong coffee in the first instance stimulates the faculties (primitive effect), but it leaves behind a sensation of heaviness and drowsiness (secondary effect), which continues a long time if we do not again have recourse to the same liquid (palliative). After exciting somnolence, or rather a deep stupor, by the aid of opium (primitive effect), it is much more difficult to fall asleep on the succeeding night (secondary effect). Constipation excited by opium (primitive effect) is followed by diarrhœa (secondary effect) ; and evacuations produced by purgatives (primitive effect) are succeeded by costiveness which lasts several days (secondary effect). It is thus that the vital power, in its re-action, opposes to the primitive effects of strong doses of medicine which operate powerfully on the healthy state of the body, a condition that is directly opposite, whenever it is able to do so.

It is only by the use of the minutest homœopathic doses, that the re-action of the vital power shows itself simply by restoring the equilibrium of health.

§ 66. But it may be readily conceived that the healthy state will make no perceptible re-action in an opposite sense, after weak and homœopathic doses of agents that modify and change its vitality. On due attention, it is true that even small doses produce primitive effects that are perceptible; but the re-action made by the living organism never exceeds the degree that is requisite for the re-establishment of health.

From these facts, the salutary tendency of the homœopathic, as well as the adverse effects of the antipathic (palliative) method, become manifest.

§ 67. These incontrovertible and self-evident truths which nature and experience have laid before us, explain, on the one hand, why the homœopathic method is so beneficial in its results, and prove, on the other, the absurdity of that which consists in treating diseases by antipathic and palliative remedies.*

* It is merely in urgent and dangerous cases, or in diseases that have just broken out in persons who were previously in health, such, for example, as in asphyxia, especially from lightning, suffocation, freezing, drowning, &c., that it is either admissible or proper, in the first instance at least, to re-animate the feeling and irritability by the aid of palliatives, such as slight electric shocks, injections of strong coffee, stimulating odours, gradual warmth, &c.** As soon as physical life is re-animated, the action of the organs that support it resumes its regular course, as is to be expected from a body that was in the full enjoyment of health previous to the accident. Under this head are also included the antidotes to several poisons, such as alkalis against mineral acids; liver of sulphur against metallic poisons; coffee, camphor (and ipecacuanha) against poison by opium, &c.

We must not imagine that a homœopathic medicine has been badly selected in a case of disease, because a few of the symptoms of this remedy correspond antipathically with some morbid symptoms of minor or less importance. Provided the other symptoms of the disease, those which are the strongest and the most developed, and finally those which characterize it, find in the remedy similar symptoms which cover, extinguish, and destroy them, the small number of antipathic symptoms that are visible disappear of themselves after the remedy has expended its action, without retarding the recovery in the slightest degree.

** And yet the new mongrel sect appeal to these remarks, though in vain, in order to find a pretext everywhere for such exceptions to the general rule, and very conveniently to introduce their allœopathic palliatives, accompanied with other mischief of a like character, merely to spare themselves the trouble of searching for suitable homœopathic remedies for every case of disease,—one might say, to save themselves the trouble of being homœopathic physicians, though they wish to be considered such. But their deeds will follow them—they are of little moment.

How far these facts prove the efficacy of the homœopathic method.

§ 68. We find, it is true, in homœopathic cures, that the

very minute doses of medicine (§ 275—287) which they require to subdue and destroy natural diseases by analogy to
the symptoms produced by the latter, leave in the organism a
slight medicinal disease which outlives the primitive affection.
But the extreme minuteness of the dose renders this disease so
slight and susceptible of dissipating itself, that the organism
has no need to oppose to it any greater re-action than that
which is requisite to raise the existing state to the habitual
degree of health—that is, to say, to establish the latter. And
all the symptoms of the primitive disease being now extinct,
a very slight effort will suffice to accomplish this (§ 65. 6.)

How these facts confirm the injurious tendency of the antipathic method.

§ 69. But precisely the reverse of this takes place in the
antipathic or palliative method. The medicinal symptom
which the physician opposes to the morbid symptom, (such as,
for example, stupefaction, which constitutes the primitive effect
of opium, opposed to an acute pain,) is not wholly foreign and
allœopathic to this latter. There is an evident affinity between
the two symptoms, but it is *inverse.* The morbid symptom is
to be annihilated here by a medicinal symptom *opposed* to it.
This cannot possibly be accomplished. It is true the antipathic remedy acts precisely on the diseased part of the organism, just as certain as the homœopathic ; but it confines itself
to covering, in a certain degree, the natural morbid symptom,
and rendering it insensible for a certain length of time. During the first moments of the action of the palliative, the organism undergoes no disagreeable sensation, neither on the
part of the morbid symptom, nor on that of the medicinal one,
which appear to be reciprocally annihilated and neutralized, as
it were, in a dynamic manner. This, for example, is what takes
place in regard to pain and the stupifying powers of opium,
for, during the first moments, the organism feels as if it were
in health, alike free from the painful sensation and the stupefaction. But as the medicinal symptom that is opposed cannot
occupy in the organism the place of the pre-existing disease,
(as is the case in the homœopathic method, where the remedy
excites an artificial disease *similar* to the natural one, but
merely *stronger,*) the vital power consequently not being affected, by the remedy employed, with a disease similar to that

which had previously tormented it, the latter does not become extinguished. The new disease, it is true, keeps the organism insensible, during the first moments, by a kind of dynamic neutralization,[1] if we may so express it, but it soon dies away of itself, like all medicinal affections ; and then it not only leaves the malady in its former state, but still more (as palliatives can never be administered but in large doses to afford apparent relief) it compels the organism to produce a state contrary to that excited by the palliative medicine, and creates an effect opposite to that of the remedy—that is to say, gives birth to a condition analogous to the natural disease, which is not yet destroyed. This addition, then, which proceeds from the organism itself, (the re-action against the palliative,) does not fail to increase the intensity and severity of the disease.[2] Thus *the morbid symptom* (this single part of the disease) *becomes worse the moment the effect of the palliative ceases, and that, too, in a degree proportionate to the extent of the dose of the palliative.* And, to continue with the same example, the greater the quantity of the opium administered to suspend the pain, in the same degree does the pain increase beyond its primitive intensity when the opium has ceased to act.[3]

[1] Contrary or opposite sensations in the living economy of man cannot be permanently neutralized like substances of opposite qualities in the laboratory of the chemist, where we may see, for example, sulphuric acid and potash form, by their union, a substance that is entirely different, a neutral salt that is no longer acid or alkali, and which not even fire will decompose. Combinations like these, producing something that is neutral and durable, can never take place in the organs of sensation with regard to impressions of an opposite nature. There is, indeed, some appearance of neutralization or of reciprocal destruction, but this phenomenon is of short duration. The tears of the mourner may cease for a moment when there is some merry spectacle before his eyes, but soon the mirth is forgotten, and the tears begin to flow again more freely than ever.

[3] However intelligible this proposition may be, it has nevertheless been misinterpreted, and an objection made to it, that a palliative would be just as well able to cure by its consecutive effect, which resembles the existing disease, as a homœopathic remedy by its primitive effect. But in raising this obstacle, it has never been considered that the consecutive effect is by no means a product of the remedy, that it always arises from the re-action exercised by the vital powers of the organism, and that consequently this reaction of the vital powers, by reason of the application of a palliative, is a state similar to the symptom of the disease which this remedy failed to anni-

hilate, and which consequently was aggravated by the re-action of the vital power against the palliative.

As in a dungeon where the prisoner scarce distinguishes the objects that are immediately before him, the flame of alcohol spreads around a consolatory light; but when the flame is extinguished, the obscurity is then greater in the same proportion as the flame was brilliant, and now the darkness that envelops him is still more impenetrable, and he has greater difficulty than before in distinguishing the objects around him.

A short analysis of the homœopathic method.

§ 70. From all that has been here stated, the following truths must be admitted :—

1st. There is nothing for the physician to cure in disease but the sufferings of the patient ; and the changes in his state of health which are perceptible to the senses—that is to say, the totality or mass of symptoms by which the disease points out the remedy it stands in need of.; every internal cause that could be attributed to it, every occult character that man might be tempted to bestow, are nothing more than so many idle dreams and vain imaginings.

2d. That state of the organism which we call disease, cannot be converted into health but by the aid of another affection of the organism, excited by means of medicines. The experiments made upon healthy individuals are the best and purest means that could be adopted to discover this virtue.

3d. According to every known fact, it is impossible to cure a natural disease by the aid of medicines which have the faculty of producing a *dissimilar* artificial state or symptom in healthy persons. Therefore the allœopathic method can never effect a real cure. Even nature never performs a cure, or annihilates one disease by adding to it another that is dissimilar, be the intensity of the latter ever so great.

4th. Every fact serves to prove, that a medicine capable of exciting in healthy persons a morbid symptom *opposite* to the disease that is to be cured, never effects any other than momentary relief in disease of long standing, without curing it, and suffers it to re-appear, after a certain interval, more aggravated than ever. The antipathic and purely palliative method is, therefore, wholly opposed to the object that is to be attained, where the disease is an important one, and of long standing.

5th. The third method, the only one to which we can still have recourse, (the homœopathic,) which employs against the totality of the symptoms of a natural disease, a medicine that is capable of exciting in healthy persons symptoms that closely resemble those of the disease itself, is the only one that is really salutary, and which always annihilates disease, or the purely dynamic aberrations of the vital powers, in an easy, prompt, and perfect manner. In this respect, nature herself furnishes the example when, by adding to an existing disease a new one that resembles it, she cures it promptly and effectually.

*The three necessary points in healing, are :—*1. *To ascertain the malady ;* 2. *The action of the medicines ; and* 3. *Their appropriate application.*

§ 71. As it is no longer doubted that the diseases of mankind consist merely of groups of certain symptoms which cannot be destroyed but by the aid of medicines, and the inherent faculty which those substances possess of exciting morbid symptoms similar to those of the natural disease, the points to be considered in the mode of treatment are the three following :—

1st. By what means is the physician to arrive at the necessary information relative to a disease, in order to be able to undertake the cure ?

2d. How is he to discover the morbific powers of medicines —that is to say, of the instruments destined to cure natural diseases ?

3d. What is the best mode of applying these artificial morbific powers (medicines) in the cure of diseases ?

A general view of acute and chronic diseases.

72. Relative to the first point, it will be necessary for us to enter here into some general considerations. The diseases of mankind resolve themselves into two classes. The first are rapid operations of the vital power departed from its natural condition, which terminate in a shorter or longer period of time, but are always of moderate duration. These are called *acute* diseases. The others, which are less distinct and often almost imperceptible on their first appearance, seize upon the organism, each according to his own peculiar man-

ner, and remove it by degrees so far from the state of health that the automatic vital energy which is destined to support the latter, and which is called vital power, cannot resist but in a useless and imperfect manner; and not being potent enough to extinguish them herself, she is compelled to allow them to grow until, in the end, they destroy the organism. The latter are known by the appellation of *chronic* diseases, and are produced by infection from a chronic miasm.

Acute diseases which are isolated—sporadic, epidemic, acute miasms.

§ 73. As to acute diseases, they may be classed under two distinct heads. The first attack single individuals, and *arise* from some pernicious cause to which they have been exposed. Immoderate excess in either eating or drinking, a want of necessary aliment, violent impressions of physical agents, cold, heat, fatigue, &c., or mental excitement, are the most frequent causes. But for the most part they depend upon the occasional aggravation of a latent psoric affection, which returns to its former sleep and insensibility when the acute affection is not too violent, or when it has been cured in a prompt manner. The others attack a plurality of individuals at once, and develop themselves here and there (*sporadically*) beneath the sway of meteoric and telluric influence, of whose action but few persons are at the moment susceptible. Nearly approaching to these are those which attack many individuals at the same time, arising from similar causes, and exhibiting symptoms that are analogous (*epidemics*); and usually become *contagious* when they act upon close and compact masses of human beings. These maladies or fevers[1] are each of a distinct nature, and the individual cases which manifest themselves being all of the same origin, they invariably place the patients everywhere in one identical morbid state, but which, if abandoned to themselves, terminate in a very short space of time, either by a cure or death. War, inundations, and famine, frequently give rise to these diseases, but they may likewise result from *acute miasms*, which always re-appear beneath the same form, for which reason they are designated by particular names; some of which attack man but once during life, such as the small-pox, measles, hooping-cough, the scarlet[2] fever of

10

Sydenham, mumps, &c.; and others which may seize him repeatedly, such as the plague, yellow-fever, Asiatic cholera, &c.

¹ The homœopathic physician, who does not share the prejudices of the ordinary schools of medicine—that is to say, who does not, like them, fix the number of those fevers to a certain few, forbidding nature to produce any others, nor affixes particular names to them in order that he may follow this or that mode of treatment—he does not acknowledge the appellations of jail fever, bilious fever, typhus, putrid fever, pituitous fever, but cures all these diseases individually by a treatment suited to the symptoms they present.

² Subsequent to the year 1801, a purple miliary fever came from the west of Europe, which physicians have confounded with scarlatina, although the signs of these two affections are entirely different, and aconite is the curative and preservative remedy of the first, and belladonna of the second, while the former always assumes the epidemic character, and the latter is mostly sporadic. Of late years, both these two affections appear to have been combined into a particular species of eruptive fever, against which neither of these two remedies were found perfectly homœopathic.

The worst species of chronic diseases are those produced by the unskilful treatment of allœopathic physicians.

§ 74. Under the class of chronic diseases, we have unfortunately to reckon those numerous factitious maladies of universal propagation, arising from the long-continued administration, by the allœopathists, of violent heroic medicines in large and increasing doses, from the abuse of calomel, corrosive sublimate, mercurial ointments, nitrate of silver, iodine and its ointment, opium, valerian, bark and quinine, digitalis purpurea, hydrocyanic acid, sulphur and sulphuric acid, long-continued evacuants, venesection, leeches, setons, issues, &c., by which the vital power is either unmercifully weakened, or, if it be not indeed exhausted, gradually becomes so abnormally altered, (in different manners, according to the particular medicine administered,) that, in order to support life against such hostile and destructive assaults, it must effect changes in the organization, and either deprive this or the other part of its sensibility or irritability, or exalt these properties to excess, produce dilatation or contraction, relaxation or induration* of parts, or else totally destroy them, and here and there induce organic changes, both internally and externally, (maim, as it were, the interior and exterior of the body,) in order to protect the organization against the entire destruction of life, from the reiterated assaults of such hostile and destructive influences.

* When, at length, the patient sinks, his physician who had prescribed such a course of treatment, takes care, on a *post mortem* examination, to exhibit to the disconsolate relatives, these internal organic arrangements (which are due to his own unskilfulness) as the original and incurable complaint.

These are the most difficult of cure.

§ 75. The most distressing and unmanageable chronic maladies affecting the human system, are those which have been superinduced by the unskilful treatment of the allœopathists, (in modern times *most injurious,) and I regret to say, that when they have attained a considerable height, it would seem as if no remedy could be discovered or devised for their cure.

It is only as there is sufficient vital power yet remaining in the system, that the injury inflicted by the abuse of allœopathic medicines can be repaired; to restore the patient, often requires a long time, and the simultaneous removal of the original malady.

§ 76. The *Dispenser of all good has granted us aid, by means of homœopathy, for the removal of natural diseases only; but those which have been superinduced by a false art —those in which the human organism has been maltreated and crippled, both internally and externally, by means of pernicious medication, the vital power itself,—provided, indeed, if it be not already too much enfeebled by such assaults, and can employ, uninterruptedly, whole years to the serious process,—the vital power must remove those factitious diseases, (assisted by appropriate aid directed against a chronic miasm, which probably still lies concealed within). An art of healing, intended for re-establishing to their normal condition those countless morbid changes of the body, which are often induced by the mischievous arts of allœopathy, does not, nor cannot exist.

Diseases that are improperly termed chronic.

§ 77. The name chronic is very improperly applied to those diseases which attack persons who are constantly exposed to baleful influences from which they might have screened themselves—persons who constantly make use of aliments or drink that are hurtful to the system—who commit excesses that are injurious to health—who are every moment in want of the articles necessary to support life—who inhabit unwholesome countries, and. above all, marshy places—who live in cellars and other confined dwellings—who are deprived of air and exercise—who are exhausted by immoderate labour of the mind or body—who are consumed by perpetual ennui, &c. These diseases, or rather these privations of health, brought on by individuals, disappear of themselves by a mere change of regimen, provided there is no chronic miasm in the body, but they cannot be called chronic diseases.

Diseases that properly claim that appellation, and which all arise from chronic miasms.

§ 78.   The true natural *chronic* diseases are those which are produced by a chronic miasm, making continual progress in the body when no specific curative remedy is opposed to them, and which, notwithstanding all imaginable care both with regard to the regimen of the body and mind, never cease tormenting the patient with an accumulation of miseries that endure till the latest period of his existence. These are the greatest and most frequent scourges of the human species, since the most robust constitution, the best regulated life, and the greatest energy of the vital powers, are insufficient to extinguish them.

Syphilis and sycosis.

§ 79.   Hitherto, syphilis only was in some measure known as one of these chronic miasmatic diseases, which, being uncured, continued to the end of life. Sycosis, which likewise cannot be subdued by the vital powers alone, has never been regarded as a distinct species of chronic disease depending on an internal miasm; and it was supposed to be cured when the excrescences on the skin were destroyed, while no attention. was paid to the source which still continued to exist.

Psora is the parent of all chronic diseases, properly so called, with the exception of the syphilitic and sycosic.

§ 80.   But a chronic miasm that is incomparably greater and far more important than either of the two last named, is that of psora. The two others disclose the specific internal affection whence they emanate—the one by chancres, and the other by excrescences in the form of a cauliflower. It is not until the whole of the organism is infected, that psora declares its huge internal chronic miasm by a cutaneous eruption (sometimes consisting only in a few pimples) that is wholly peculiar to it, accompanied by insupportable tickling, voluptuous itching, and a specific odour. This psora is the sole true and fundamental cause that produces all the other countless forms of disease* which, under the names of nervous debility, hysteria, hemicrania, hypochondriasis, insanity, melancholy, idiocy, madness, epilepsy, and spasms of all kinds, softening of the bones, or rickets, scoliasis and cyphosis, caries, cancer, fungus hæmatodes, pseudomorphæ of all kinds, gravel, gout, hæmorrhoids, jaundice and cyanosis, dropsy, amenorrhea, gastrorrhagia, epistaxis, hemoptysis, hematuria; metrorrhagia, asthma and phthisis ulcerosa, impotency and sterility, deafness, cataract and amaurosis, paralysis, loss of sense, pains of every kind, &c., appear in our pathology as so many peculiar, distinct, and independent diseases.

* It has cost me twelve years of study and research to trace out the source of this incredible number of chronic affections—to discover this great truth which remained concealed from all my predecessors and cotemporaries—to establish the basis of its demonstration, and find out, at the same time, the principal antipsoric remedies that were fit to combat this hydra in all its different forms. My observations on this subject have been given to the world in the *Treatise on Chronic Diseases* which I published in the year 1828–30, iv. vols. Dresden, by Arnold. (Second edition. 1835.) Until I had examined the depths of this important matter, it was impossible for me to teach the mode of subduing all chronic diseases but as isolated and individual affections by the medicinal substances that were till then known according to their effects upon healthy persons; so that the followers of my method treated each case of chronic disease separately as a distinct group of symptoms, which, however, did not prevent their cure to such an extent that suffering humanity had good cause to rejoice at the newly-discovered system of medicine. But how much more satisfactory must it be, now that remedies have been discovered which are still more homœopathic for the cure of chronic diseases that owe their origin to psora! from among which the physician, who is truly skilled in his art, will select only such whose medicinal symptoms correspond best with those of the chronic disease which it is intended to cure.

§ 81. The progress of this ancient miasm through the

organisms of millions of individuals in the course of some hundreds of generations, and the extraordinary degree of development which it has by these means acquired, will explain, to a certain extent, why it is able at present to make its appearance beneath so many different forms, especially if we contemplate the multiplicity of circumstances[1] that usually contribute to the manifestation of this great diversity of chronic affections, (secondary symptoms of psora,) besides the infinite variety of their individual constitution. It is, therefore, not surprising that such different organisms, penetrated by the psoric miasm, and exposed to so many hurtful influences, external and internal, which often act upon them in a permanent manner, should also present such an incalculable number of diseases, changes, and sufferings, as those which have, till the present time, been cited by the old pathology[2] as so many distinct diseases, describing them by a number of particular *names.*

●

[1] Some of these causes, which, in modifying the manifestation of psora, give to it the form of a chronic disease, evidently depend, in a certain degree, either on climate and the natural situation of the dwelling, or on the diversities of the physical and moral education of youth, which has, in some instances, been either neglected or too long delayed, and in others carried to excess, or on the abuse of it in respect to regimen, passions, morals, customs, and habits.

[2] How many are found among them whose names bear more significations than one, and by each of which very different diseases are designated, that have no connection with each other but by a single symptom! Such as *ague, yellow jaundice, dropsy, phthisis, leucorrhœa, hæmorrhoids, rheumatism, apoplexy, spasms, hysteria, hypochondriasis, melancholy, insanity, angina, paralysis,* &c., (☞ in this country, *dyspepsia, liver complaint, disease of the spine,* and other fashionable terms,) which are represented as fixed diseases that always preserve their identity, and which, by reason of the name they bear, are always treated upon the same plan. How can we justify the identity of medical treatment by the adoption of a name! And if the treatment is not always to be the same, why make use of an identical name, which also supposes a coincidence in the manner of being attacked by medicinal agents! *Nihil sane in artem medicam pestiferam magis unquam irrepsit malum quam generalia quædam nomina morbis imponere iisque aptare velle generalem quandam medicinam :* it is thus that Huxham, a physician as enlightened as he is admired for his candour, has expressed himself. (Op. Phys. Med. t. i.) Fritze likewise complains (Annalen, i. p. 80) that the same names have been given to diseases that are essentially different.

Even epidemic diseases, which are probably propagated by a specific miasm in each particular case of epidemy, receive names from the existing medical school, as if they were fixed diseases, already known and always returning under the same form. It is thus they speak of *hospital fever, jail fever, camp fever, bilious fever, nervous fever, mucous fever,* &c., although each epidemic of these erratic fevers manifests itself beneath the aspect of a new disease that never existed before, varying considerably both in its course and in the most characteristic symptoms, and also in its whole department. Each of them differs so widely from all the anterior epidemics, whatever names they bear, that it is overturning every principle in logic to give to diseases so manifestly different from each other, one of those names that have been introduced into the pathology, and then to regulate the medical treatment according to a name that has been so abused. Sydenham alone discovered the truth of this (Oper. cap. 2, de morb. epid. p. 43) ; for he insists upon the necessity of never believing in the identity of one epidemic disease with another that had manifested itself before, or of treating it according to this affinity, because the epidemics which exhibit themselves successively have all differed from each other. *Animum admiratione percellit, quam discolor et sui plane dissimilis morborum epidemicorum facies ; quæ tam aperta horum morborum diversitas tum propriis ac sibi peculiaribus symptomatis, tum etiam medendi ratione, quam hi ab illis disparem sibi vindicant, sqtis illucescit. Ex quibus constat morbos epidemicos, utut externa quatantenus specie et symptomatis aliquot utrisque pariter convenire paullo incautioribus videantur, re tamen ipsa, si bene adverteris animum alienæ esse admodum indolis et distare ut æra lupinis.*

From all this, it is clear that these useless names of diseases, which are so much abused, ought to have no influence whatever upon the plan of treatment adopted by a true physician who knows that he is not to judge of and treat diseases after the nominal resemblance of a symptom, but according to the totality of the signs of the individual state of each patient; his duty is, therefore, to search scrupulously for diseases, and not to build his opinion upon gratuitous hypotheses.

Should it, however, be thought sometimes necessary to have names for diseases in order to render ourselves intelligible in a few words to the ordinary classes when speaking of a patient, let none be made use of but such as are collective. We ought to say, for example, that the patient has a species of chorea, a species of dropsy, a species of nervous fever, a species of ague, because there certainly do not exist any diseases that are permanent and always retaining their identity, which deserve these denominations or others that are analogous. It is thus we might by degrees dissipate the illusion produced by the names given to diseases.

Every case of chronic disease demands the careful selection of a remedy from among the specifics that have been discovered against chronic miasms, particularly against psora.

§ 82.　Although the discovery of this great source of chronic affections has advanced the science of medicine some steps

nearer to that of the nature of the greater number of diseases
that present themselves for cure, still the homœopathic physician, at every chronic disease (psoric) that he is called upon
to treat, ought not to be less careful than before in seizing
upon the perceptible symptoms, and everything that is connected with them; for it is no more possible in these diseases
than in others to obtain a real cure without particularizing
each individual case in a rigorous and absolute manner. It
is only necessary to distinguish whether the disease is acute
or chronic, because, in the first case, the principal symptoms
develop themselves more rapidly, the image of the malady is
found in a much shorter time, and there are far fewer inquiries to be made, because the greatest part of the signs are of
themselves more evident to the senses* than is the case in
chronic diseases of several years' standing, whose symptoms
are ascertained with greater difficulty.

* According to this, the method I am about to point out for the discovery of the symptoms is only suited in a partial degree to acute diseases.

Qualifications necessary for comprehending the image of the disease.

§ 83. This examination of a particular case of disease,
with the intent of presenting it in its formal state and indi-
viduality, only demands, on the part of the physician, an unprejudiced mind, sound understanding, attention and fidelity
in observing and tracing the image of the disease. I will content myself, in the present instance, with merely explaining
the general principles of the course that is to be pursued,
leaving it to the physician to select those which are applicable to each particular case.

*Direction to the physician for discovering and tracing out an image of the
disease.*

§ 84. The patient details his sufferings; the persons who
are about him relate what he has complained of, how he has
behaved himself, and all that they have remarked in him.
The physician sees, hears and observes, with his other senses,
whatever there is changed or extraordinary in the patient.
He writes all this down in the very words which the latter,
and the persons around him, made use of. He permits them

to continue speaking to the end without interruption,* except where they wander into useless digressions, taking care to exhort them at the commencement, to speak slowly, that he may be enabled to follow them in taking down whatever he deems necessary.

* Every interruption breaks the chain of ideas of the person who speaks, and things do not afterwards return to his memory in the same shape he would at first have described them.

§ 85. At each new circumstance related by the patient or e ersons present, the physician commences another line, in order that the symptoms may all be written down separately, and stand one beneath the other. By this mode of proceeding, he will be enabled to add to that which has, in the first instance, been related to him in a vague manner, anything he may subsequently acquire from a more accurate knowledge of the case.

§ 86. When the patient and those about him have finished all they had to say, the physician then asks for more precise information with regard to each individual symptom, and proeds as follows :—He reads over all that has been communicated to him, and asks at each particular symptom, for example—At what epoch did this or that circumstance occur? Was it previous to the use of the medicines which the patient has taken till the present time, or while he was taking them, or only a few days after he had discontinued their use? What kind of pain, what particular sensation was it that was felt in such or such a part of the body? Which the precise spot that it occupied? Did the pain come on in separate attacks at intervals, or was it lasting and uninterrupted? How long did it continue? At what hour of the day or night, and in what part of the body was it most violent, or where and when did it cease entirely? What was the precise nature of this or that particular circumstance or symptom?

§ 87. Thus the physician causes all the indications which were given in the first instance to be described to him more closely, without ever appearing, by his manner of putting the question, to dictate the answer,* or place the patient in such a position that he shall have nothing to reply but yes or no to his

question. To act otherwise would only lead the person interrogated to deny or affirm a thing that is false, or only half
true, or even wholly different from that which has really occurred, according as it may suit his convenience, or for the purpose of gratifying the physician. An unfaithful description of
the disease would then result, and, consequently, an inappropriate choice of the curative remedy.

* For instance, the physician ought never to say—" Did not such or such
a thing take place in this manner ?" By giving this turn to his questions,
he puts a false reply into the mouth of the patient, and draws from him a
wrong indication.

§ 88. If in this spontaneous narrative no mention is made
of several parts or functions of the body, and of the state of
mind of the patient, the physician may then ask if there is not
something more to be said respecting this or that particular
part or function, or relative to the disposition and state of
mind,† taking care, at the same time, to confine himself to
general terms, in order that the person who furnishes the explanation may, thereby, be constrained to answer categorically
upon these various points.

† For example—Has the patient had an evacuation from his bowels ?
How does he pass water—freely or otherwise ? How does he rest by day
and by night ? What is the state of mind and temper of the patient ? Is he
thirsty ? What kind of taste has he in the mouth ? What kinds of food and
drink are most agreeable to him, and which are those he dislikes ? Do the
different articles taste as usual, or have they another taste that is wholly different ? How does he feel after meals ? Have you anything more to tell me
relative to the head, belly, or limbs ?

§ 89. When the patient (for it is to him we are to refer, in
preference, for everything that relates to the sensations he experiences, except in diseases where concealment is observed)
has thus personally given the necessary details to the physician,
and furnished him with a tolerable image of the malady, the
latter is then at liberty to question him more specifically
if he finds he is not yet sufficiently informed on the subject.*

* For example—How often have the bowels been evacuated, and what was
the nature of the discharges ? Did the whitish discharges consist of mucus
or fæces ? Were they painful or otherwise ? What was the precise nature
of these pains, and in what part were they felt ? What did the patient throw
up ? Is the bad taste in the mouth putrid, bitter, or acid, or what kind of

taste is it? Does he experience this taste before, during, or after eating or drinking? At what part of the day does he feel it in particular? What kind of taste was connected with the eructation? Is the urine turbid at first, or does it only become so after standing awhile? Of what colour was it at the time of emission? What was the colour of the sediment? Is there any peculiarity in the state of the patient when he sleeps? Does he sigh, moan, speak, or cry out? Does he start in his sleep? Does he snore in inspiration or expiration? Does he lie on his back only, or on which side does he lay himself? Does he cover himself up close, or does he throw off the bed-covering? Does he easily awake, or does he sleep too soundly? How does he feel on waking? How often does this or that symptom occur, and on what occasion? Is it when the patient is sitting up, lying down, standing up, or when he is moving about? Does it come on merely when he has been fasting, or at least early in the morning, or simply in the evening, or only after meals, or if at other times, when? When did the shivering come on? Was it merely a sensation of cold, or was he actually cold at the time? In what part of the body did the patient feel cold? Was his skin warm when he complained of being cold? Did he experience a sensation of cold without shivering? Did he feel heat without the face being flushed? What parts of his body were warm to the touch? Did the patient complain of heat without his skin being warm? How long did the sensation of cold, or that of heat, continue? When did the thirst come on? During the cold or heat? Or was it before or after? How intense was the thirst? What did the patient ask for to drink? When did the perspiration come on? Was it at the commencement or at the expiration of the heat? What space of time elapsed between the heat and the perspiration? Was it when sleeping or waking that it manifested itself? Was it strong or otherwise? Was the perspiration hot or cold? In what parts of the body did it break out? How did it smell? What did the patient complain of before or during the cold, during or after the heat, during or after the perspiration, &c.?

§ 90. All the answers being committed to writing, the physician then notes down what he himself observes in the patient,* and endeavours to ascertain if that which he observes existed or not when the latter was in health.

* For example—How he behaved during the time of the visit? Was he irritable, peevish, quarrelsome, hasty, grieved, anxious, despairing, sad, calm, or resigned? Did he appear overcome with sleep, or lost in reverie? Was he hoarse? Did he speak low? Was his discourse incoherent, or how was it? Of what colour was the countenance, the eyes, and the skin, generally? What degree of vivacity was there visible in the face and eyes? How was the tongue, the respiration, the smell from the mouth, or the hearing? Were the pupils of the eyes dilated or contracted? Did they contract and dilate quickly in light and darkness, and in what degree? What was the state of the pulse? What was the condition of the abdomen? Was the skin moist and warm, cold or dry, upon this or that part of the body, or was it so all

over ! Did the patient lie with his head thrown back, with his mouth wholly or half open, with his arms crossed above his head; was he on his back, or in what position was he ! Did he raise himself with difficulty ! In short, the physician is to keep notes of everything he has observed that is strange and remarkable.

§ 91. The symptoms which appear, and the sensations of the patient during the use of medicine or shortly after, do not furnish a true image of the disease. On the contrary, the symptoms ând the inconveniences which exhibited themselves *previous to the use of the medicines*, or *several days after their discontinuance*, give the true fundamental notion of the *original* form of the malady. These are, therefore, to be noted down in preference by the physician. When the disease is of a chronic nature, and the patient has already made use of reme- dies, he may be allowed to remain some days without giving him any medicine, or at least without administering anything but substances that are not medicinal. A rigorous examina- tion may likewise be deferred for the same space of time, because it is the means of obtaining permanent symptoms in all their purity, and of being able to form a true representation of the disease.

§ 92. But where an acute disease is to be treated, so dan- gerous in its nature as not to admit of delay, and the physician can learn nothing of the symptoms that manifested themselves previous to the remedies, then he is to view the whole of the existing symptoms as they have been modified by the latter, in order that he may at least be able to seize upon the present state of the disease; that is to say, be enabled to embrace in one and the same image the primitive disease and the medici- nal affection conjointly. The latter of these being most fre- quently rendered more severe, and at the same time more dangerous than the former, by the application of remedies that are generally the very opposite of those which ought to have been administered, they often demand immediate assistance, and the prompt application of the appropriate homœopathic remedy, in order to prevent the patient falling a sacrifice to the irrational treatment he has undergone.

§ 93. If the acute disease has been caused recently, or if the chronic one has been so for a longer or shorter period of time by some remarkable event, and if the patient or the parents, when interrogated secretly, do not disclose this cause, the physician must then use his address and prudence in order to arrive at a knowledge of it.*

* Should there be anything humiliating in that which has given birth to the disease, so that the patient, or those about him, hesitate in avowing the cause, or at least in declaring it spontaneously, the physician ought then to seek to discover it by questions that are skillfuly turned, or by secret inquiries. In the catalogue of these causes are ranked, poisoning or attempts to commit suicide, onanism, ordinary or unnatural debauchery, excesses at table, or in the use of wine, cordials, punch, and other spirituous drinks, riotous eating generally, or especially unwholesome food, venereal or psoric affection, disappointed love, jealousy, domestic disappointments, anger, grief occasioned by a family misfortune, bad treatment, repressed vengeance, injured pride, embarrassment in pecuniary affairs, superstitious fear, famine, defect of the organs of reproduction, hernia, prolapsus, &c.

§ 94. On inquiry into the state of a chronic disease, it is requisite to weigh the particular circumstances in which the patient may be placed in regard to ordinary occupation, mode of life, and domestic situation. All these circumstances ought to be examined, to discover if there is any thing that could give birth to and keep up the disease, so that by its removal the cure may be facilitated.*

* By chronic diseases in the female sex, it is, above all, necessary to pay attention to pregnancy, sterility, amorous desire, accouchement, miscarriage, lactation, and the state of the catamenia. As regards the latter, it is always necessary to ask if it returns at too short intervals, or at others that are too distant, how long it continues, if the blood flows uninterrupted or only at intervals, if the flow is copious, if it be of a dark colour, if leucorrhœa appears before or after ; what is the state of the body and mind previous to, during, and subsequent to the menses ; if the female is attacked with leucorrhœa, of what nature it is ; in what quantity does it appear, and under what circumstances, and on what occasion did it manifest itself.

§ 95. In chronic affections, the symptoms before enumerated, and every other appertaining to the malady, ought to be examined as rigorously as possible, going into all their minutiæ. In short, it is in these diseases that they are most developed, and least resemble those of acute affections ; they also require to be studied with the utmost care if the treatment is to succeed. On the other hand, the patients are so accustomed to their long sufferings, that they pay little or no attention to the lesser symptoms which are often very characteristic of the dis-

ease, and decisive in regard to the choice of the remedy ; they
look upon them as though they were in a manner belonging to
their physical state, and constituted a part of that health, the
real sentiment of which they had forgotten during the fifteen
or twenty years their sufferings have endured, and never entertain a suspicion that there can be any connection between
these symptoms and the principal disease.

§ 96. Added to this, the patients themselves are of such
very opposite tempers, that some, particularly the so called
hypochondriacs, and others who are sensitive and impatient,
depict their sufferings in lively colours, and make use of
exaggerated terms to induce the physician to relieve them
promptly.*

* Even the most impatient hypochondriac never invents sufferings and
symptoms that are void of foundation, and the truth of this is easily ascertained by comparing the complaints he utters at different intervals while the physician gives him nothing at least which is medicinal ; it is merely requisite to
retrench a part of his exaggeration, or at least ascribe the energy of his expressions to his excessive sensibility. In this respect, even the exaggeration he is guilty of in describing his sufferings becomes an important
symptom in the list of those which constitute the image of the disease. It is
a very different case with maniacs, and those who feign disease through
wickedness or other causes.

§ 97. Others, on the contrary, either through indolence, mistaken modesty, or finally by a sort of mildness and timidity,
are silent with regard to many of the sufferings they endure,
and only hint at them in obscure terms, or point at them as
being of little importance.

§ 98. If it be then true that we are to rely more particularly
upon the patient's own language in describing his sufferings
and sensations, and prefer the expressions he makes use of to
portray them (because his words are almost always changed
in passing through the mouths of those who are about him) ;
it is no less so, that in all diseases, and more especially in those
of a chronic character, the physician must be possessed of an
uncommon share of circumspection and tact, a knowledge of
the human heart, prudence and patience, to be enabled to form
to himself a true and complete image of the disease in all its
details.

§ 99. The examination into acute diseases, or those that have recently broken out, is generally less difficult, because the patient and those about him are struck with the difference between the existing state of things and the health that has been so recently destroyed, of which the memory still retains a lively image. Here, also, the physician must necessarily be acquainted with every thing; but there is less occasion for being urgent in acquiring the particulars, which, for the most part, come before him spontaneously.

Investigation of epidemic diseases in particular.

§ 100. With regard to a search after the totality of the symptoms in epidemic and sporadic diseases, it is wholly indifferent whether anything similar ever existed before in the world or not, under any name whatever. Neither the novelty nor the peculiarity of an affection of this kind will make any difference in the mode of studying it, or in that of the treatment. In fact, we ought to regard the pure image of each prevailing disease as a thing that is new and unknown, and study the same from its foundation, if we would really exercise the art of healing—that is to say, we ought never to substitute the hypothesis in the room of the observation, never regard any given case of disease as already known, either in part or wholly, without having first carefully examined all its appearances. This prudent mode of proceeding is so much the more requisite here, as every reigning epidemic is, in many respects, a particular species of phenomenon, and which, upon attentive examination, will be found to differ greatly from all former epidemics to which the same has been wrongfully applied. We must, however, except those epidemics which are caused by miasm that always retain their identity, such, for example, as the measles, small-pox, &c.

§ 101. It may happen that a physician, who, for the first time, treats a person attacked with an epidemic disease, will not immediately discover the perfect image of the affection, because a knowledge of the totality of the signs and symptoms in these collective maladies is not acquired till after having observed several cases. However, a practised physician will, after having treated one or two patients, see so far into the real state of things as to be often able to form to himself a characteristic image of the same, and know what homœopathic remedy he is to have recourse to, in order to combat the disease.

§ 102. By carefully noting down all the symptoms observed in several cases of this description, the image that has once been formed of the malady will be always rendered still more comprehensive. It neither becomes extended in a greater degree, nor lengthened in the detail, but it is made more graphic and characteristic of the peculiarities of the collective malady. On the one side, the general symptoms (such, for example, as loss of appetite, insomnolency, &c.) acquire a still greater degree of precision ; on the other, the special and more marked symptoms, which are even rare in epidemics, and belong elsewhere to a small number of diseases only, develop themselves and form the character of the disease.* It is true, that persons attacked with an epidemic have all a disease arising from the same source, and consequently equal ; but the entire extent of an affection of this nature, together with the totality of the symptoms—a knowledge of which is necessary to form a complete image of the morbid state, and to choose according to that the homœopathic remedy most in harmony with the *ensemble* of the symptoms—cannot be observed in the case of a single patient ; in order to arrive at these, it will be requisite to abstract them from a view of the sufferings of several patients of different constitutions.

* The physician who has already in a first case discerned an approximate homœopathic remedy, will, by a study of successive ones, be enabled to prove whether the choice he made was appropriate, or this will point out to him a remedy that is still more suitable than the former, or even one that is better than all others.

In like manner must the source of chronic disease (not syphilitic) be investigated, and the entire image of psora brought into view.

§ 103. In the same manner as is here taught in reference to epidemic, and chiefly acute diseases, I·had to investigate those of a miasmatic and chronic character, (always remaining identical in their nature,) and particularly psora. This examination was conducted with much more accuracy than had hitherto been observed, in order to grasp the disease in its entire compass, since different patients are affected with dissimilar symptoms, and each particular case embraces but one disjointed part, as it were, of the symptoms constituting the totality of one and the same disease. Hence it is manifest, that the totality of the symptoms appertaining to such a chronic malady, to psora in particular, could only be collected by the examination of numerous individual patients, and without obtaining an entire view, and forming a collective image of that malady, the medicines (viz. the antipsorics) which are efficient for its entire removal, and which, at the same time, are the true remedies for the particular cases of it, could not be discovered.

The utility of noting down in manuscript the image of the disease at the commencement and during the progress of the treatment.

§ 104. The totality of the symptoms which characterize a given case—or, in other terms, the image of the disease—being once committed to writing, the most difficult part is accomplished.* The physician ought ever after to have this image before his eyes to serve as a basis to the treatment, especially where the disease is chronic. He can then study it in all its parts, and draw from it the characteristic marks, in order to oppose to these symptoms—that is to say, to the disease itself—a remedy that is perfectly homœopathic, whose choice has been decided on according to the nature of the morbid symptoms which it produces from its simple action on the body. And if, during the course of the treatment, he inquires after the effects of the remedy, and the changes that have taken place in the state of the patient, it only remains to obliterate from the group of primitive symptoms those which have entirely disappeared, to note down those of which there are still some remains, and add the new ones which have supervened.

* The physicians of the old school, in their treatment of the sick, adopt an extremely convenient method. No accurate inquiries are heard from them concerning all the circumstances of the case; and the patients, during the recital of their individual symptoms, are not unfrequently interrupted by the physician to prevent disturbance in the rapid writing of his prescriptions, compounded of a medley of ingredients, the genuine effects of which are unknown to him. No allœopathic physician, as already observed, desires to know a full and accurate account of the symptoms, much less to commit them to writing. If after several days he re-visits his patient, (numerous others having been seen in the interval,) he will then have retained in his memory

11

little or nothing of the minute circumstances of the case, as at first heard, and
what had passed into one ear will have escaped from the other. In his succeeding visits, he does little more than ask a few general questions, feels the
pulse, looks at the tongue, and forthwith, without an intelligible reason, proceeds to write another prescription, or directs the former (in large and frequently repeated portions through the day) to be continued. Then with mien
polite he hastens to the fiftieth or sixtieth patient of those whom he has visited
in the same thoughtless manner on the same day. Thus a profession which,
of all others, properly requires the most reflection, the conscientious and
careful examination of each and every case, and the special cure founded
thereon,—such a profession is thus practised by persons who call themselves
rational physicians.

*Preliminaries to be observed in investigating the pure effects of medicines in
the healthy human subject. Primary effect. Secondary effect.*

§ 105. The *second point* in the duty of the physician is to
examine into the instruments destined to cure natural diseases, to
study the morbific powers of medicines, in order, when he is
to cure a disease, that he may be able to find one among the
number whose list of symptoms constitutes a factitious disease
that resembles as closely as possible the principal signs of the
natural malady which he intends to cure.

§ 106. It is necessary to know the full extent of the power
by virtue of which each medicine excites a disease. In other
terms, it is requisite that all the morbid symptoms and changes
of the health which their action individually is capable of producing in the economy shall have been observed, as closely as
possible, before any one can hope to be able to find or select
from among them homœopathic remedies that are appropriate
to the greater number of natural diseases.

§ 107. If, to arrive at this object, we were only to administer medicines to *invalids,* prescribing them, one by one, in a
simple state, little or nothing would be seen of their pure
effects, because the symptoms of the natural disease then existing mingling with those which the medicinal agents are
capable of producing, the latter can rarely be distinguished
with any clearness or precision.

§ 108. Thus there is no safer or more natural method of
discovering the effects of medicines on the health of man, than
by trying them separately and singly, in moderate doses, upon

healthy individuals, and observing what changes they create in the moral and physical state ; that is to say, what elements of disease these substances are capable of producing :* for, as we have before seen, (§ 24—27,) the entire curative virtues of medicines depend solely upon the power they have of modifying the state of health, which is illustrated by observing the effects resulting from the exercise of this faculty.

* In the course of twenty-five centuries, no physician, that I know of, except the immortal Haller, has ever thought of a method so natural—so absolutely necessary, and so perfectly true—as that of observing the pure effects of each medicine individually, in order to discover, by that means, the diseases they were capable of curing. Before me, Haller was the only one who conceived the necessity of pursuing such a plan (see the preface to his Pharmacopœia Helvet. Basil, 1771, p. 12). " *Nempe primum in corpore sano medela tentanda est, sine peregrina ulla miscela; odoreque et sapore ejus exploratis, exigua illius dosis ingerenda et ad omnes, quæ inde contingunt, affectiones, quis pulsus, quis calor, quæ respiratio, quænam excretiones, attendendum. Inde ad ductum phænomenorum, in sano obviorum, transeas ad experimenta in corpore ægroto,*" &c. But no physician has profited by this invaluable advice ; no one has paid the slightest attention to it.

§ 109. I am the first who has pursued this path with a perseverance that could alone result from, and be supported by, the intimate conviction of this great truth so valuable to the human race,[1] that the homœopathic administration of medicines is the sole certain method of curing disease.[2]

[1] It is as impossible that there should be any other true method of curing dynamic diseases (*i. e.* those not surgical) besides homœopathy, as that more than one straight line can be described between two given points. How little can they be grounded in the true art of healing, who imagine that there is yet another way of curing diseases, who, after having thoroughly contemplated the basis of homœopathy and practised it with sufficient care, or, from upright motives, have either read of or witnessed homœopathic cures, and, on the other hand, duly weighed the groundlessness of every species of allœopathic treatment, and inquired into the sinister effects thence arising— who, with a loose indifference, place upon an equality the true art of healing with that injurious method, or pronounce it the sister of homœopathy, whose company she cannot dispense with! My conscientious successors, the genuine and accurate adherents of homœopathy, who have practised it with almost infallible success, could teach them a better lesson.

[2] The first fruits of my labours, so far as they could then be perfected, are contained in a work entitled Fragmenta de viribus medicamentorum positivis, sive in sano corp. hum. observatio, p. i. ii. Leipsic, 1805, in 8vo. Others, that are still more matured, are contained in the two editions of my Materia

Medica, (*Reine Arzneimittellehre*, 6 vols. in 8vo., third edition, 1833,) and in the second and following volumes of my Treatise on Chronic Diseases. *Die Chronische Krankheiten. Dresden*, 1828, in 8vo. second edition, 1835.

§ 110. On perusing the works of authors who have written upon the morbid effects caused by medicinal substances, which, through negligence, mischief, criminal intent, or otherwise, had got into the stomachs of healthy individuals in large quantities, I saw that the facts they contained coincided with the observations which I had made in trying them on myself and other persons in health. These are reported as cases of poisoning, and as proofs of the inherent pernicious effects of these energetic agents, pointing out the danger of making use of them. By some, they have been mentioned for no other purpose than that of making a parade of the skill they manifested in the discovery of remedies which gradually restored the health of persons that otherwise would have been lost by such violent means. Others, to free their consciences of the death of patients, have alleged the malignity of these substances which they then designated poisons. Not one among them has ever suspected that the symptoms, in which they wished merely to see proofs of the poisonous qualities of drugs which produce them, were certain indications that disclosed the existence in these identical substances of the faculty of annihilating (under the title of remedies) similar symptoms in natural diseases. No one imagined that the evils which they excite were so many certain proofs of their homœopathic effects. They never imagined that an observance of the changes to which medicines give birth in healthy persons was the sole means of discovering their medicinal and curative virtues, because they can neither arrive at this result by any specious reasoning *à priori*, nor by the smell, taste, or appearance of the medicinal substances, nor by chemical analysis, nor by administering prescriptions to patients where they are associated with a less or greater number of other drugs. Finally, none of them ever had the slightest presentiment that these histories of diseases produced by medicine would one day furnish the elements of a true and pure materia medica— a science which, from its origin down to the present time, has consisted of a mass of false conjectures and fictions, or which, in other terms, never yet had any real existence.*

* See what I have said on this subject in my " Treatise on the Sources of the ordinary Materia Medica," in the third part of the " Reine Arzneimittellehre."

§ 111. The conformity of my observations upon the pure effects of medicines with those of a more ancient date, which were made without reference to any curative aim, and even the correspondence of these latter with others of a similar kind that are spread throughout the writings of various authors, plainly prove to us that medicinal substances, in creating a morbid state in healthy persons, follow *fixed and eternal laws of nature,* and are, in virtue of those laws, severally capable of producing, (*each according to its own peculiar properties,*) *certain positive morbid symptoms.*

§ 112. In the descriptions that have been handed down to us by early writers of the frequent dangerous consequences resulting from the administration of medicines in large doses, symptoms have also been remarked that did not show themselves at the beginning of these sad events, but merely towards the conclusion, and which were perfectly opposite to those at the commencement. These symptoms, contrary to the *primitive effect* (§ 63), or to the so called action of medicines on the body, are owing to the re-action of the vital force of the organism. They constitute the *secondary* and *consecutive effect* (§ 62—67), whose traces are seldom perceived when moderate doses, by way of trial, are employed ; and when the doses are small, no vestige ever remains, because in homœopathic cures the living organism never re-acts beyond what is absolutely necessary to bring the disease back to the natural state of health (§ 67).

§ 113. Narcotic substances, alone, are exceptions to this rule. As they, in their primitive effects, extinguish sensibility, sensation, and irritability, to a certain extent, it often happens that when they are tried on healthy persons, even in moderate doses, they have the secondary effect of exciting the sensibility and increasing the irritability.

§ 114. But with the exception of narcotic substances, all medicines that are tried in small doses, upon healthy persons, only manifest their primitive effects; that is to say, the symptoms which indicate that they modify the habitual state of

health, and excite a morbid condition which is to last for a
longer or shorter period.

Alternative effects of medicines.

§ 115. Among the primitive effects of some medicines, there
are several to be found that are contrary, or at least in certain
respects, accessory, to other symptoms which afterwards appear in succession. This circumstance, however, is sufficient
to make us regard them as so called *consecutive effects*, or as a
simple result of the re-action of the organism. They merely
mark the transition from one to the other of the different paroxysms of the primitive action. They are called *alternative*
effects.

Idiosyncrasies.

§ 116. Certain symptoms are excited by medicines more
frequently than others—that is to say, in many patients ; some
are more rarely produced, and in a small number of persons,
while yet others are only so in a few individuals.

§ 117. To these last belong the so called *idiosyncracies*, by
which are meant particular constitutions, which, though in
other respects healthy, yet have a tendency to be placed in a
greater or less morbid state by certain things that do not *appear* to make any impression on many other persons, or cause
any change in them.' But this absence of effect upon such or
such an individual is only so in appearance. In short, as the
production of every morbid change whatever pre-supposes the
faculty of action in the medicinal substance, and in the patient that of being affected by it, the manifest changes of
health that take place in idiosyncracies cannot be wholly attributed to the particular constitution of the patient. It is necessary to ascribe these, at the same time, to the things that
have given them birth, and which embrace the faculty of exercising the same influence over all men, with this exception,
that among healthy persons there are but a small number who
have a tendency to allow themselves to be placed in so decided a morbid condition. What proves that these agents
really make an impression upon all individuals is, that they
cure homœopathically in all patients the same morbid symp-

toms as those which they themselves appear to excite only in persons subject to idiosyncrasies.[2]

[1] The smell of the rose will cause certain persons to faint; others are sometimes attacked with dangerous diseases after eating muscles, crabs, or the fry of the barbel, and after touching the leaves of a certain species of sumac.

[2] Thus the Princess Maria Porphyrogeneta restored her brother, the Emperor Alexius, suffering from syncope, by sprinkling him with rose water, (τὸ τῶν ῥόδων στάλαγμα), in the presence of her aunt, Eudoxia, (Hist. Byz. Alexias, lib. 15, p. 503, ed. Posser.,) and Horstius, (Oper. iii. p. 59,) saw that vinegar of roses was very helpful in syncope.

Every medicine produces effects different from others.

§ 118. Each medicine produces particular effects in the body of man, and no other medicinal substance can create any that are precisely similar.*

* This fact was also recognised by Haller, who says, (in the preface to his Hist. Stirp. Helv.,) "Latet immensa virium diversitas in iis ipsis plantis, quarum facies externas dudum novimus, animas quasi et quodcunque cœlestius habent, nondum perspeximus."

§ 119. In the same manner that each species of plant differs from all others in its external form and peculiar mode of vegetation—its smell and taste; in the same manner that each mineral and each salt differs from others in regard to external character as well as internal chemical properties, (a circumstance which alone ought to have sufficed to prevent confusion,) in the same manner do all these substances likewise differ from each other in regard to their morbific effects, and, consequently, their curative powers.[1] Each substance exercises upon the health of man a certain and particular influence which does not allow itself to be confounded with any other.[2]

[1] He who knows that the action of each substance upon the body differs from that of every other, and who can appreciate the importance of this fact, will have no difficulty in discovering that there can be no such things (in a medical point of view) as succedanea—that is to say, medicines that are equivalent, and capable of replacing each other mutually. It is only he who is ignorant of the certain and pure effects of medicinal substances, that can be so foolish as to endeavour to persuade us that one remedy can serve in the room of another, and produce the same salutary effect in any given case of disease. In this manner children, through their simplicity, confound things that are

essentially different, because they hardly know them otherwise than by their exterior, and have no idea of their innate properties or of their real intrinsic value.

* If this be the pure truth, as it undoubtedly is, then can no physician who wishes to preserve a quiet conscience, and to be looked upon as a reasonable man, henceforward prescribe any other medicines than those with whose true value he is precisely and thoroughly acquainted—that is to say, those whose action upon healthy individuals he has studied with sufficient attention to be convinced that any particular one among them was that which, of all others, produced the morbid state most resembling the natural disease it was intended to cure ; for, as we have before seen, neither man nor nature ever effects a perfect, prompt, and durable cure, but by the aid of a homœopathic remedy.   No physician can, therefore, in future, disregard a research of this nature, without which it would be impossible for him to acquire the knowledge of medicines indispensable to the exercise of his art, which has been neglected till the present time.   Posterity will scarcely believe that, until th' present day, physicians have always contented themselves with administe' ing blindly in disease, remedies of whose real value they were ignora' whose pure and dynamic effects, upon healthy persons, they had never s died, and that they were in the habit of mixing several of those unkno' substances whose action is so diversified, and then left it to chance to d. pose of whatever might accrue to the patient from this treatment.   It is ii this manner that a madman, who has just forced his way into the workshop of an artist, seizes with open hands upon all the tools within his reach for the purpose of finishing a work which he finds in a state of preparation.   Who can doubt but that he will spoil it by the ridiculous manner in which he goes to work, or perhaps even destroy it entirely?

Every medicine must therefore be carefully tried as to the peculiarities of its effects.

§ 120.   Thus we ought to distinguish medicines carefully one from another, since it is on them that life and death, disease and health, depend.   To effect this, it is necessary to have recourse to pure experiments, made with care, for the purpose of developing the properties that belong to them, and the true effects which they produce on healthy individuals. By this mode of proceeding we may learn to know them properly, and so avoid their misapplication in the treatment of disease ; for nothing but a judicious choice of the remedy that is to be employed can ever restore to the patient, in a prompt and permanent manner, that supreme of all earthly blessings —a sound mind in a healthy body.

Course to be adopted in trying medicines upon other individuals.

§ 121.   In studying the effects of medicines upon healthy persons, it must not be forgotten that even the administration of moderate doses of the so called heroic remedies is sufficient to produce modifications in the health of the most robust individuals. Medicines that are more gentle in their nature ought to be given in larger doses if we would likewise prove their action. Finally, if we would try the effects of the weakest substances, the experiment must be made upon persons only who are, it is true, free from disease, but who, at the same time, are possessed of a delicate, irritable, and sensitive constitution.

§ 122. In circumstances of this nature, on which depend the certitude of the medical art, and the welfare of future generations, it is necessary to employ only medicines that are well known, such as we are convinced remain pure, unadulterated, and possessed of their full energy.

§ 123. Each of these medicines ought to be taken in its simple and pure form. As to indigenous plants, the juice is expressed and mixed with a small quantity of alcohol, in order to preserve it from corruption. With regard to foreign plants, they are to be pulverized or prepared as spirituous tinctures, and mixed with a certain quantity of water previous to administration. Salts and gums, however, ought not to be dissolved in water till the moment they are to be used. If a plant cannot be procured but in its dry state, and if its powers are naturally feeble, it may be tried in the form of an infusion; that is to say, after having cut it up small, boiling water is poured upon it, in order to extract its virtues. The infusion ought to be drunk immediately after its preparation, and while it is still warm, because all the juices of plants, and all vegetable infusions to which no alcohol is added, pass rapidly into fermentation and corruption, and thereby lose their medicinal virtues.

§ 124. Every medicinal substance that is submitted to a trial of this nature ought to be employed alone, and perfectly pure. Care must be taken not to add any heterogeneous substance to it, or to use any other medicine, either on the same day and much less on those that follow, if we would observe the effect it is capable of producing.

§ 125.   During the whole time of this experiment the diet must be extremely moderate.   It is necessary to abstain as much as possible from spices, and to make use of nothing but simple food that is merely nourishing, carefully avoiding all green vegetables,[1] roots, sallads, and soups with herbs, all of which, notwithstanding the preparations they have undergone, are aliments that still retain some small medicinal energy that disturbs the effect of the medicine.   The drink is to remain the same as that in daily use, taking care that it is as little stimulating as possible.[2]

[1] Green peas, French beans, and even carrots, may be allowed, as being vegetables that contain the least medicinal properties.
[2] The subject of experiment must either have been previously unaccustomed to the use of wine, ardent spirits, coffee, or tea, or have for some time thoroughly abstained from these stimulating and medicinally injurious beverages.

§ 126.   The person on whom this experiment is tried ought to avoid all fatiguing labour of mind and body, all excesses, debauches, or mental excitement, during the whole of the time that it continues.   No urgent business must prevent him making the necessary observations, and he must of his own accord be scrupulously attentive to everything that passes in the interior of the body without permitting anything to interrupt his care, and finally, unite with a healthy body (in its kind) a necessary degree of judgment, that he may be able to express and describe clearly all the sensations he experiences.

§ 127.   Medicines should be tried on the persons of women as well as of men, in order that those changes in the economy which are referable to difference of sex, may be clearly ascertained.

§ 128.   The most recent experience has taught that medicinal substances, when taken by the experimenter in their crude state for the purpose of testing their peculiar effects, do not for a long time display the full extent of those virtues which lie concealed within them, as is the case when they are taken in higher developments, i. e., exalted in power by due trituration and agitation.   By means of this simple mode of preparation, the virtues which, in the crude state of the medicines, lay concealed, and, as it were, dormant within them, become incredibly developed and aroused into activity. Thus, any one even of those medicines whose virtues are considered weak, is now found to be the most advantageously investigated, if from four to six minute saccharine globules impregnated with the thirtieth (decillionth) dilution of such medicine, and mixed with a little water, be given to the experimenter every morning, fasting, and continued for several days.

§ 129. When the effects of one such dose appear to be weak, then it may be daily increased a few globules, until the effects become stronger and more distinct, until the changes in the system be evident, for one particular medicine does not affect every individual in a like manner, or with the same degree of energy ; on the contrary, there exists, in this respect, the greatest diversity possible. Sometimes a person apparently delicate is not at all affected by a medicine that is known to be very powerful, though administered in moderate doses, while other substances that are much weaker make a tolerable impression on him. At the same time, there are individuals of robust constitutions who experience very considerable morbid symptoms from medicinal agents that are apparently mild, and, on the other hand, they are likewise but little affected by others that are powerful. But as it can never be known beforehand which of these two cases will occur, it is proper that each should commence with a small dose, and be afterwards increased progressively, if deemed requisite ; advancing, from day to day, to higher and still higher doses.

§ 130. If at the commencement, and after administering the first dose, the effects are sufficiently powerful, one advantage results from it, which is, that the person who undergoes the experiment becomes acquainted with the succession of symptoms which this agent principally excites, and is enabled to note them down with precision the moment they appear, a circumstance of vast import to a knowledge of the character of medicines, because the order of their primitive effects, and likewise that of their alternative effects, is thus exhibited in the

least equivocal manner. A very weak dose often suffices, if
the individual on whom it is tried is endowed with great sensibility, and pays due attention to his state. The length of time
that the action of a medicine continues, can only be known by
a comparison of the results of several experiments.

§ 131. If, to acquire at least some knowledge of a medicine,
it is found requisite to administer to the same person, several
days in succession, doses of the same, progressively increased,
this may show us the various morbid changes that this substance is capable of exciting generally ; but we do not learn
the order of their succession, and a succeeding dose often extinguishes one or other of the symptoms produced by the preceding one, or creates in its place a contrary state. Symptoms
of this kind should be noted between two parentheses, as being
equivocal, until new experiments of a purer nature shall have
decided whether they are to be considered as the re-action of
the organism, or the alternative effects of the medicine.

§ 132. But where it is intended merely to find out what are
the symptoms that a medicinal substance, particularly a weak
one, is capable of producing by itself, without paying any
attention to the order of these symptoms, or to the duration of
the action of the medicine, it is advisable to continue the experiment several days successively, only augmenting the dose
each day. By this means, the effects of even the most gentle
medicines that are unknown will come to light, particularly if
they are tried on a sensitive person.

§ 133. Should the individual who undergoes the experiment
experience any particular inconvenience from the action of the
medicine, it is useful, and even necessary, to the exact determination of the symptom, that he should place himself successively in various postures, and observe the changes that ensue.
Thus he will be enabled to examine whether the motion
communicated to the suffering parts by walking up and
down the chamber, or in the open air, seated, lying down, or
standing, has the effect of augmenting, diminishing, or dissipating the symptom, and if it returns or not upon resuming the
original position. He will also perceive whether it changes
when he eats or drinks, or by any other condition, when he

speaks, coughs, or sneezes, or in any other action of the body whatsoever. He must also observe at what hour of the day or night the symptom more particularly manifests itself. All these details are requisite, in order to discover what is peculiar and characteristic in each symptom.

§ 134. All external agents, particularly medicines, produce changes in the state of the living organism that vary each in themselves. But the whole of the symptoms peculiar to any medicinal substance whatever, never manifest themselves in the same individual, neither do they appear simultaneously, or during a single experiment ; on the contrary, the same person experiences, in preference, at one time, one set of symptoms, and in a second or third experiment yet others, (with another person these or other symptoms will appear,) so that by the fourth, eighth, or tenth person, perhaps, some or more of the symptoms which had already manifested themselves in the second, sixth, ninth, &c., will be visible. Neither do the symptoms re-appear at the same hour.

§ 135. It is only by repeated observations made upon a great number of individuals of both sexes, properly selected for the purpose from among a variety of constitutions, that we can acquire a pretty accurate knowledge of the whole of the morbid effects that a medicine is capable of producing. There can be no certainty of having properly proved the symptoms of any medicinal agent—that is to say, of the faculty which it has of changing the health, until such time as the persons who make further trials of it perceive but few new symptoms arising from its use, and observe almost always only those that have been previously remarked by other persons.

§ 136. Although, as before stated, the medicine that is tried upon a healthy person cannot manifest on a single individual all the modifications of health which it is capable of producing, and only exhibits them in several persons, differing from one another in regard to physical constitution and moral disposition, it is, however, equally true, that the eternal and immutable law of nature has endowed it with the faculty of exciting these symptoms in every human being (§ 117). This is the cause of all its effects, of even those which it is rarely

seen to produce in healthy persons, but which do not fail to
appear when administered to a patient attacked with a disease
resembling the one it is capable of exciting. Provided the
medicine be homœopathically chosen, and administered even
in the smallest doses possible, it will then produce in the
patient an artificial state approaching closely to the natural
disease, and cure the latter in a prompt and durable manner.

§ 137. The more moderate the dose, (without, however,
going beyond a certain limit,) the more are the primitive
effects developed which are most important to be known.
Scarcely any but the latter will then be perceptible, and there
will be hardly any traces of re-action. But it is understood
that the individual on whom the experiment is made must be
one who can be relied upon in regard to veracity—that he is
moderate in every respect, of a sensitive mind and body, and
shall attend to his person with all possible care. On the other
hand, if the dose be excessive, there will not only be several
re-actions visible among the symptoms, but yet more, the
primitive effects will manifest themselves in a manner so precipitate, violent, and confused, that it will be impossible to
make any correct observation. Let us add to this, the danger
that might result from it to the individual on whom the experiment is tried, which cannot be regarded as a matter of
indifference by one who has any respect for his fellow-mortals,
and who looks upon every human being in the light of a
brother.

§ 138. Provided all the conditions before stated (§ 124—
127) (which are necessary to the trial of a pure experiment)
be complied with, the symptoms, modifications, and changes
of the health that are visible during the action of the medicine, depend upon that substance alone, and ought to be noted
down as properly belonging to it, if even similar symptoms,
occurring spontaneously, should have been experienced *a long
time before* by the person on whom the experiment is made.
The re-appearance of those symptoms, in the course of the
experiment, only proves that in virtue of his own constitution
this person has a special tendency to admit of their manifestation. In this case, they are the effects of the medicine, for it
cannot be said that they came of themselves at a moment

when a powerful medicinal agent exercised its sway over the entire organism.

§ 139. Where the physician does not try the remedy on his own person, and the experiment is made on another individual, it is requisite for the latter to note down, with perspicuity, all the sensations, inconveniences, symptoms, and changes, that he experiences at the very moment of their occurrence. He must also be able to tell what time elapsed between the administration of the medicine and the appearance of each symptom, and in case they continued any length of time, what was the exact period of their duration. The physician is to read this report, immediately after it is finished, in the presence of the person on whom the experiment is made ; or if it lasts several days, he then reads it over each day, in order that, by refreshing his memory, the person may be enabled to reply to the questions which it may be necessary to put to him relative to the precise nature of each symptom, and to give him an opportunity of adding fresh details, or making any necessary corrections.*

* He who publishes to the medical world such experiments, is responsible for the credibility of the experimenter, as well as for the correctness of his statements, and very properly so, as the welfare of suffering humanity is at stake.

§ 140. If the individual cannot write, the physician must then interrogate him each day, in order to learn his sensations. But this examination ought, for the most part, to be confined to listening to his narrative. The physician must not indulge in any conjectures or suppositions, and he is to ask as few questions as possible, taking care to maintain the same circumspection and reserve, which I have before recommended (§ 84—99), as an indispensable precaution in seeking the information requisite to form the image of the natural disease.

The experiments which a physician in health makes in his own person are preferable to others.

§ 141. But of all the pure experiments relative to the changes which simple medicines produce, and the morbid symptoms they excite in healthy persons, those are always the best which a physician (enjoying a good state of health, free

from prejudice, and able to analyze his sensations) makes on
his own person, observing, at the same time, the precautions
that have just been prescribed.   A thing is never more certain than when it has been tried on ourselves.*

* The experiments that are made on our own persons have one advantage
above all others.   In the first place, they furnish a conviction of this great
truth, that the curative virtues of medicines depend solely upon the power
they possess of creating changes in the physical economy of man.   In the
second place, they teach us to understand our own sensations, mind, and disposition, which is the source of all true wisdom, (γνῶϑι σεαυτὸν,) and exercise
our powers of observation, an indispensable talent in a physician.   All our
observations on others are by no means so interesting as those made on ourselves.   In all the observations made on other individuals, it is continually
to be feared that the person making trial of the remedy may not exactly
experience that which he says, or will not express in a proper manner that
which he feels.   The physician must always remain in doubt, or at least
partly so, whether he is deceived or not.   This obstacle to a knowledge of
the truth, which cannot be entirely obviated in a search after the morbid
symptoms excited in another person by the action of the remedy, does not
exist where the trial is made on our own persons.   The individual who undergoes the experiment knows precisely what he feels, and every fresh
attempt that he makes is an additional motive for him to extend his researches
still farther, by directing them towards other remedies.   It renders him more
expert in pursuing farther trials, while at the same time his zeal is redoubled,
because he thereby acquires a true knowledge of the resources of the art,
which can be considerably increased.   Do not let him suppose, on the other
hand, that the slight inconveniences which he subjects himself to in trying
the medicines on his own person can be detrimental to his health.   On the
contrary, experience has shown us that they only render the body more apt
to repel all natural and artificial morbific causes, and harden it against their
influence.   The same experience also teaches, that thereby the health
becomes more firm, and the body more robust.

*The investigation of the pure effects of medicines by their administration in
disease, is difficult.*

§ 142.   But how the symptoms,* produced by a simple
medicine, can be distinguished among the symptoms of the
original disease, even in those which mostly retain their identity, more especially chronic diseases, is an object for superior
discernment, and to be left to masters in observation.

* Symptoms which had been remarked only a long time before, if at all
throughout the whole course of the disease, and which, of course, are new
ones, and are the product of the medicine.

It is by investigating the pure effects of medicines in the healthy subject only, that a true materia medica can be framed.

§ 143. After having thus tried a number of simple medicines upon the healthy body, faithfully and carefully noting all the symptoms they are capable of producing as artificial morbific agents, then only can we acquire a true materia medica —that is to say, a catalogue of the pure and certain effects of medicinal substances. This will furnish us with a code of nature, in which will be inscribed, from every agent so investigated, a considerable number of particular symptoms, as they were manifested to the observation of the experimenter; among these, are the (homœopathic) morbid elements resembling those of several natural diseases which are hereafter to be cured by them; in a word, they comprehend artificial morbid states which supply, for the similar morbid states naturally induced, the only true, homœopathic, *i. e.* specific instruments of certain and permanent cure.

§ 144. A materia medica of this nature shall be free from all conjecture, fiction, or gratuitous assertion—it shall contain nothing but the pure language of nature, the results of a careful and faithful research.

§ 145. We ought certainly to be acquainted with the pure action of a vast number of medicines upon the healthy body, to be able to find homœopathic remedies against each of the innumerable forms of disease that besiege mankind—that is to say, to find out artificial morbific powers that resemble them.[1] But thanks to the truth of the symptoms, and to the multitude of morbid elements which each of the energetic medicines that have been tried till the present day upon healthy persons have exhibited, there now remain but few diseases against which we do not find in these substances suitable homœopathic remedies,[2] which restore health in a gentle, certain, and permanent manner. An infinitely greater number of diseases are cured by these means, and in a far safer and more certain manner, than by a treatment guided by the general and special therapeutics of allœopathy, with all its unknown and mixed medicines, which only alter and impair, but cannot cure, chronic diseases, and rather retard than promote recovery from those that are acute.

12

[1] At first I was the only individual who made it a chief and important study to find out the principal and pure effects of medicines. But what cures shall we not be able to perform in the vast empire of disease, when numerous observers,[**] upon whose accuracy and veracity we can rely, shall have contributed the result of their researches (trials on their own persons) to enrich this materia medica, the only one that is founded on fact. The art of curing will then approach to the same degree of certainty as the science of mathematics.

[1] See the third note to § 109.

[**] Among the remedies which have been tried more particularly, the following were at first introduced :

1. *By Hahnemann.*—Aconitum, alumina, amanita, ambra, ammoniæ carbonas, angustura, argentum, arnica, arseniosum acidum, artemisia santonica, asarum, aurum; barytæ carbonas, belladonna, bismuthi subnitras, bryonia; calcis carbonas, calcis sulphuretum, camphora, cannabis, cantharis, capsicum, carbo animalis, carbo vegetabilis, causticum, chamomilla, chelidonium, cicuta, cinchona, cocculus, colocynthis, conium, copaiva, cyclamen; digitalis, drosera, dulcamara; euphrasia; ferrum; graphiles, guaiacum; helleborus, hydrarg. solub., hydrarg. corros., hyoscyamus; iodium, ipecacuanha; ledum, lycopodium; magnes. carb., magnes. mur., manganum, menyanthes, moschus, mur. acidum; nitri acidum, nux vomica; oleander, opium; petroleum, phosphorus, phosphoric. acid., potassæ carbonas, pulsatilla; rheum, ruta; sambucus sassaparilla, scilla, sepia, silica, sodæ carbonas, sodii chloretum, spigelia, spongia, stannum, staphisagria, stramonium, sulphur, sulphuric acid.; taraxacum, toxicodendron, thuya; veratrum, verbascum, viola tricolor.

2. By *Stapf.*—Agnus, anacardium, antimonii et potassæ tartras; barytæ acetas; clematis, coffea, colchicum; euphorbium; lamium; marum verum; mezereum; paris.; sabadilla, sabina.

3. By *Gross and Stapf.*—Crocus; platina.

4. By *Gross.*—Epeira; sodæ nitras;.viola odorata.

5. By *Franz.*—Assa fœtida; cuprum; ranunculus; veleriana; zincum.

6. By *Hartlaub.*—Æthusa, antimon. sulphuretum; bovista; cantharis; gratiola; indigo; krameria; laurocerasus; oleum animale; phellandrium, phosphorus, plumbum, potassæ iodidum; strontianum; tabacum, terebinthi oleum.

7. By *Hering.*—Arum; brucea; caladium, curcas; jambos; lachesis et crotalus; phosphas calcis, psorinum; selenium, sericum, solanum mammosum; theridion; urea.

8. By *Heine.*—Actæa, alkekengi, aquilegia; chenopodium, chiococca; nigella.

9. By *Nenning*—Ammoniæ murias; magn. sulphas, millefolium; niccolum; sodæ sulphas; tongo.

10. By *Caspari.*—Castoreum; terri oxyd. magneticum.

11. By *Wahle.*—Laurocerasus; prunus spinosa.

12. By *Seidel.*—Rhododendron; senega.

13. By *Schreter.*—Potassæ nitras; sodæ boras.

14. a, By *Apel.*—Amanita. b, *Attomyr.*—Corallia. c, *Bute.*—Rhus vernix. d, *Helbig.*—Myristica. e, *Hesse.*—Berberis. f, *Trinks.*—Secale.

At the same time, while making trials, they mutually assisted each other, and had help from many others, so that, in addition to the names above given, we find mentioned among those who tried them, the following: Ahner, Adams, Becher, Bethman, Baehr, Behlert, Bauer, Becker, Cubitz, Flämming, Freitag, Gatmann, Gersdorff, Fr. Hahnemann, Hartmann, Haubold, Hromada, Hempel, Hornburg, Hugo, Haynel, Ihm, Kummer, Langhammer, Lehmann, Lingen, Matlack, Meyer, Michler, Müller, Pleyel, Preu, Th. and L. Rückert, Rummel, Rosazewsky, Romig, Reichhelm, Schoenke, Sonnenberg, Schweickert, Schmid, Schmoele, Teuthorn, Tieze, Wagner, Wislicenus, Wesselhöft, De Yöung; and a great many individuals participated, more or less, some handing in their names, and others contributing anonymously.   C. Hg.

The most appropriate remedial employment of medicines whose peculiar effects are known.

§ 146. The *third point* in the duty of a physician is to *employ* those medicines whose pure effects have been proved upon a healthy person in the *manner best suited to the cure of natural diseases homœopathically.*

That medicine which is the most homœopathically adapted, is the most bene- ficial, and is the specific remedy.

§ 147. Of all these medicines, that one whose symptoms bear the greatest resemblance to the totality of those which characterize any particular natural disease, ought to be the most appropriate and certain homœopathic remedy that can be employed ; it is the specific remedy in this case of dis- ease.

Intimation how a homœopathic cure is probably effected.

§ 148. A remedy which has the power and tendency to produce an artificial disease closely resembling the natural one against which it is employed, and which is administered in proportionate doses, affects, in its action on the organism, precisely those parts which had till then been a prey to the natural disease, and excites in them the artificial disease which it is naturally capable of producing. The latter, by reason of its similitude and greater intensity, now substitutes itself for the natural disease. From that moment it then re- sults that the vital powers no longer suffer from the last men- tioned, which, in its quality of purely dynamic immaterial power, has already ceased to exist. The organism is no longer attacked but by the medicinal disease. But the dose of the remedy administered having been very small, the med- icinal disease soon disappears of itself. Subdued by the energy of the vital power, like every other mild medicinal affection, it leaves the body free from suffering—that is, in a perfect and permanent state of health.

The homœopathic cure of a disease of rapid origin is quickly effected, but the cure of a chronic one requires proportionably a longer time.

§ 149. When a proper application of the homœopathic remedy has been made,* the acute disease which is to be

cured, however malignant and painful it may be, subsides in
a few hours, if recent, and in a few days, if it is somewhat
older. Every trace of indisposition vanishes; scarcely anything is seen of the artificial disease produced by the remedy;
and health is restored by a speedy and almost insensible transition. Diseases that are of long standing, especially those
which are complicated, require a longer treatment. Particularly those chronic artificial maladies which the maltreat-
ment of the allœopathists so often produce, and which, along
with the uncured natural disease, requires a far longer time
for recovery; they are often nearly incurable, by reason of
the shameless deprivation of the vital energies of the patient,
the prevailing and principal measure adopted by the allœopathists is their so called cures.

* But the difficult and sometimes very laborious affair of searching out and
selecting the homœopathic medicine, which shall be adapted in all respects
to the morbid conditions of a given case, is one which, notwithstanding all
the praiseworthy attempts to simplify the labour by adminiculary publications,
requires the study of the sources themselves, besides the exercise of much
circumspection and deliberation, which meet with their best recompense in
the consciousness of having faithfully performed our duties. But how will
this careful and laborious process, by which the best cure of diseases can
only be effected, please the gentlemen of the new mongrel sect, who, while
pluming themselves with the honourable title of homœopathists, for appearance' sake, administer a medicine in the form of homœopathic, that they have
hastily snatched up (*quidquid in buccam venit*). If it does not immediately
relieve, they will not impute the failure to their own unpardonable indolence
and levity in hurrying over one of the most important and critical of human
concerns, but to homœopathy,—they reproach its imperfections, because it
does not of itself, without any trouble on their part, provide the suitable
homœopathic remedy, and, as it were, serve it up like food already cooked,
and prepared to their hands. They know, indeed, full well how to console
themselves for the failure of their scarcely half homœopathic remedy, by
dexterously calling in requisition the more pliable resources of allœopathy,
whence a few dozen of leeches are applied, or a small and harmless venesection
of eight or ten ounces is prescribed in due form; and if, after all, the patient
should recover, they extol the leeches and the venesection, &c., as if he
would not have recovered without them. They cause it to be understood
in no equivocal language, that, without the trouble of racking their brains,
these operations afforded by the pernicious routine of the old school would,
in truth, have been the best means of cure. If, however, the patient should
sink under the treatment, they endeavour to soothe the disconsolate relatives
by declaring "that they themselves were witnesses, how that everything
imaginable had been done for the deceased!" Who would honour such a

light-minded and pernicious sect, by calling them, after the difficult yet beneficent art, homœopathic physicians?

Slight indisposition.

§ 150. If a patient complain of slightly accessory symptoms, which have just appeared, the physician ought not take this state of things for a perfect malady that seriously demands medicinal aid. A change in the diet and mode of life usually suffices to remove so slight an indisposition.

Severe diseases exhibit a variety of symptoms.

§ 151. But if the few symptoms of which the patient complains are very violent, the physician who attentively observes him will generally discover many others which are less developed, and which furnish a perfect picture of the malady.

A disease with numerous and striking symptoms, admits of finding the homœopathic remedy with more certainty.

§ 152. The more intense an acute disease, the more evident and numerous are its symptoms, while at the same time it is also easy to discover suitable remedies, provided there is a sufficient number of medicines to select from, whose positive action on the body is known. Among the symptoms produced by a great number of medicines, it is easy to find one that contains morbid elements, from which might be composed an artificial disease very similar to the totality of the symptoms of the natural disease that is present. This is precisely the remedy that is desirable.

What kind of symptoms ought chiefly to be regarded in selecting the remedy.

§ 153. In searching after a homœopathic specific remedy —that is to say, in making a comparison of the entire symptoms of the natural disease with those produced by known remedies, in order to discover among the latter an artificial morbific power resembling the natural disease that is to be cured—we ought to be particularly and almost exclusively attentive to the symptoms that are *striking, singular, extraordinary*, and *peculiar*, (characteristic,)* *for it is to these latter*

that similar symptoms, from among those created by the medicine, ought to correspond, in order to constitute it the remedy
most suitable to the cure.   On the other hand, the more vague
and general symptoms, such as loss of appetite, headache,
weakness, disturbed sleep, uncomfortableness, &c., merit little
attention, because almost all diseases and medicines produce
something as general.

* The most complete work extant for showing the various effects which
medicinal agents produce, and their correspondence with the various maladies they are capable of removing, is Jahr's Manual of Homœopathic Medicine, translated from the German, with improvements and additions, by C.
Hering, M. D., Allentown.—EDITOR.

A remedy that is perfectly homœopathic, cures the disease without any accompanying ill effects.

§ 154.   The more this counter representation, formed from
the symptoms of the medicine which appear to deserve a preference, sha l contain other symptoms resembling those which
are extraordinary, peculiar, and characteristic, in the natural
disease, the greater will be the resemblance on either side,
and the more homœopathic, suitable, and specific, will this
medicine be in the present case.   A disease that is of no very
long standing ordinarily yields, without any great degree of
suffering, to a first dose of this remedy.

The reason why homœopathic cures are thus effected.

§ 155.   I say *without any great degree of suffering*, because
when a perfect homœopathic remedy acts upon the body, it is
nothing more than symptoms analogous to those of the disease labouring to surmount and annihilate these latter by
usurping their place.   The remaining symptoms, caused by
the medicinal substance, which are often numerous, and correspond in no respect with the existing malady, scarcely ever
show themselves, and the patient improves from hour to hour.
The reason of this is, that the dose of any medicine applied
homœopathically being necessarily very feeble, this substance
does not possess sufficient power to exhibit its effects non-
homœopathically in the parts of the body that are free from
disease.   But it produces its effects homœopathically in those
parts of the organism that are already a prey to the irritation

arising from the symptoms of the natural disease, and excites in them a stronger medicinal affection which extinguishes and annihilates the other.

Reason of the few exceptions thereto.

§ 156. There is no homœopathic remedy, however suitably chosen, that does not (especially in a dose not small enough) produce at least during its action some slight inconveniences or fresh symptoms in very sensitive and irritable patients. In fact, it is scarcely possible for the symptoms of the medicine to cover those of the malady with as much precision as a triangle would do in regard to another which is possessed of angles and sides that are equal to its own. But these differences, which are of little importance in a case that terminates in a short time, are easily effaced by the energy of the vital principle, and the patient does not perceive it himself, unless he is excessively delicate. The re-establishment of health goes forward, notwithstanding, unless impeded by the influence of heterogeneous medicinal agents upon the patient, errors of regimen, or excitement of the passions.

The medicinal disease, closely resembling, but rather more intense than the primitive one, called also homœopathic aggravation.

§ 157. But although it is certain that a homœopathic remedy, administered in a small dose, quietly annihilates the acute disease which is analogous to it without producing its other non-homœopathic symptoms—that is to say, without exciting new and grievous sufferings; it often happens, notwithstanding, that it produces, at the expiration of one or a few hours after ingestion, (according to the dose,) a state something less favourable, which resembles the primitive affection so closely that the patient supposes the original disease aggravated. But in reality it is nothing more than a *medicinal disease*, extremely similar to the primitive one, and rather more intense in its nature.

§ 158. This trifling *homœopathic aggravation* of the malady during the first few hours—this happy omen which announces that the acute disease will soon be cured, and that it will, for the most part, yield to a first dose—is perfectly as it ought to be, because the medicinal disease should naturally be rather more intense than the one it is intended to cure, if it is to sub- due and extinguish the latter; in the same way as a natural disease can destroy another that resembles it, by exceeding it in power and intensity, (§ 43—48.)

§ 159. The smaller the dose of the homœopathic remedy, the slighter the apparent aggravation of the disease, and it is proportionably of shorter duration.

§ 160. As a homœopathic dose, however, can scarcely ever be made so small as not to amend, and, indeed, perfectly cure and destroy the undisturbed, natural disease, analogous to it, and of recent origin, (§ 249, note,) it may be readily conceived wherefore a suitable homœopathic remedy, if not given in the very smallest dose, should always occasion, in the first hour after its administration, a remarkable homœopathic aggrava- tion of this nature.*

* This preponderance of the symptoms of the remedy over those of the analogous symptoms of the disease, which looks like an increase of the nat- ural malady, has also been observed by other physicians when chance led them to a homœopathic medicine. When the patient, afflicted with itch, after having taken sulphur, complains that the cutaneous eruption grows worse, the physician, who is ignorant of the cause, consoles him by saying that the itch comes out entirely before it can be cured; but he is not aware that it is an exanthema caused by the sulphur, which assumes an appearance of aggravated itch.

Leroy (Med. Instr. for Mothers) informs us that the *viola tricolor* com- menced its action by rendering the cutaneous eruption of the face worse, of which it subsequently effected the cure; but he did not know that the appa- rent increase of the evil was caused solely by the administration of too large a dose of the remedy, which, in this instance, turned out to be homœopathic. Lysons (Medic. Trans. vol. ii. London, 1772) says, that the skin diseases which yield with the greatest certainty to elm bark are those which it in- creases in the first instance. If he had not, according to the prevailing cus- tom of the allœopathic school, administered the bark of the elm in too large doses, but if, as its homœopathic character requires, it had been given in extremely small doses, the exanthemata against which he prescribed it would have been cured without experiencing this increase of intensity, or, at least, they would have been subjected to but a very slight development.

In chronic (psoric) diseases, the aggravation produced by homœopathic reme- dies, (antipsorics,) occurs from time to time for several days.

§ 161. When I fix the so-called homœopathic aggravation (or rather the primitive action of the homœopathic remedy

which appears in a slight degree to increase the symptoms of
the natural disease) to the first hour or the first few hours, this
delay applies to acute affections that have recently intervened.* But when the remedies whose action lasts for a long
time have to combat a disease of some duration, or one of
very long standing, and consequently the dose ought to continue its action several days successively, then we may see,
during the first six, eight, or ten days, from time to time, some
of those apparent aggravations of the original malady which
last during one or several hours, while the general amendment
develops itself sensibly in the intervals. When these few days
are once passed, the amelioration produced by the primitive
effects of the remedy continues, without interruption, for some
days longer.

* Although the effects of remedies whose action is of the longest duration
rapidly disappear in acute diseases, they last a considerable time in chronic
affections ; (arising from psora ;) and thence it occurs that antipsoric remedies
do not often produce this slight homœopathic aggravation of the symptoms
during the first hours, but bring it on later and at different periods during the
first eight or ten days.

*Measures to be pursued in the treatment, when the number of known medi-
cines is too small to admit of finding a remedy that is perfectly homœopathic.*

§ 162. *The number of medicines whose pure and precise action is known being moderate* (200), it sometimes happens, that
only a part of the symptoms of the disease that is to be cured
are to be found among those of the most homœopathic remedy,
and, consequently, this imperfect remedy is obliged to be employed for want of another that is less so.

§ 163. In this case, a perfect cure, free from all inconvenience on the part of the remedy employed, ought not to be
expected. During its use, some symptoms are seen to appear
that were not observed before in the disease ; these are accessory symptoms resulting from a medicine that is not perfectly
homœopathic with the existing case. This does not, however,
prevent the remedy from annihilating a great part of the evil
—that is to say, the morbid symptoms which resemble those of
the medicinal disease, and thence arises a tolerable commencement towards a cure.

§ 164. The small number of homœopathic symptoms in a

well-selected homœopathic remedy, never injures the cure *when it is in a great measure composed of the extraordinary symptoms which particularly distinguish and characterize the disease ;* the cure then follows without further inconvenience to the patient.

§ 165. But if among the symptoms of the remedy not one is to be found that bears a perfect resemblance to the striking and characteristic symptoms of the malady—if the totality of them does not correspond with this latter, but in regard to general symptoms that are badly developed, (nausea, faintness, headache, &c.)—and among the known medicines there is not one to be found more homœ pathic, or which could be selected for the purpose—the physician ought not to expect an immediate favourable result from the administration of a remedy so imperfectly homœopathic.

§ 166. This is, however, *very rarely* the case, particularly as the number of medicines whose pure effects have been discovered is considerably increased of late ; and when it does occur, the inconveniences that flow from it are diminished after another remedy is employed, whose symptoms bear a yet greater resemblance to those of the malady.

§ 167. In short, if the application of an imperfect homœopathic remedy used, in the first instance, causes any accessory symptoms of some importance, the action of the first dose is not allowed to exhaust itself in acute diseases ; the altered state of the patient is then to be examined, and the remainder of the primitive symptoms to be joined to those which have been recently discovered, to form of the whole a new image of the disease.

§ 168. A remedy that is analogous may then be easily found among the medicines that are known, a single application of which will suffice, if not to destroy l e disease entirely. at least to facilitate the cure in a great degree. If this new remedy is not sufficient to restore the health completely, then examine what yet remains of the diseased state, and select the homœopathic remedy that is most suitable to the new image that results from it. In this manner the physician must continue until he attains his object—that is to say, until he has fully restored the health of the patient.

§ 169. It may easily occur, on examining a disease for the first time, and also on selecting for the first time the remedy that is to combat it, that the totality of the symptoms of the disease is found not to be sufficiently covered by the morbific symptoms of a single medicine, and that two remedies dispute the preference as to the eligibility in the present instance, the one being homœopathic to one part of the disease, and the other still more so to another. It is then by no means advisable, after using the preferable of the two remedies, to take the other without examination, because the medicine given as the inferior of the two, under the change of circumstances, may not be proper for the remaining symptoms; in which case, it follows that a suitable homœopathic remedy should be selected for the new set of symptoms in its stead.

§ 170. In the present instance, as well as in every other where a change has taken place in the state of the disease, it is requisite to seek out what actually remains of the symptoms, and select as suitable a remedy as possible to the present state of the malady, without any reference whatever to that one which, in the commencement, appeared to be the second best of the two remedies that were found suitable. Should it still happen, though it is not often the case, that the medicine which at first appeared as the second best, may now be very suitable to the rest of the morbid symptoms, it will then be the more worthy of confidence, and should be used in preference.

§ 171. In non-venereal chronic diseases, (consequently those which owe their origin to psora,) it is often necessary in the cure to employ several remedies one after the other, each of which ought to be chosen homœopathic to the group of symptoms which still exist after the preceding one has exhausted its action; and which may have been applied in a single dose, or in several in succession.

Measures to be taken in the treatment of diseases that have too few symptoms,
(Einseitige Krankheiten.)

§ 172. The *small number of symptoms in disease* gives rise to another *difficulty* in the cure—a circumstance which has an equal claim to our attention, since by its removal we do

away with nearly all the obstacles that this system presents;
for, if we except the yet incomplete apparatus of known
homœopathic remedies, this is the most perfect of all curative
methods.

§ 173. The only diseases that appear to have but few
symptoms, and which are, therefore, more difficult to cure, are
those which may be called *partial* (*einseitige*), because they
have but one or two principal and prominent symptoms which
mask almost all the others. These are for the most part
chronic diseases.

§ 174. Their principal symptom is, perhaps, either an
internal malady, (such, for example, as cephalalgia, diarrhœa,
cardialgia, &c.. of long standing,) or a more external injury.
These latter affections, particularly, are called *local diseases*.

§ 175. As to partial diseases of the first species alluded to,
the want of attention on the part of the physician is frequently
the reason that he does not fully trace out the symptoms which
are extant, by whose aid he would be able to form a more
complete outline of the image of the disease.

§ 176. There are, however, some few diseases which, notwithstanding all the care with which they may be examined
in the first instance, (§ 84—98,) exhibit only one or two strong
and violent symptoms, while all the others are manifest but
in a slight degree.

§ 177. A case of *this description very rarely* occurs; but
when it does, it will be requisite, in a successful treatment, to
commence by selecting, according to the indication of the few
symptoms that are perceptible, that medicine which appears
to be the most homœopathic.

§ 178. It sometimes may happen that this remedy, carefully
selected according to the exigency of the homœopathic law,
will present the artificial disease, which, by its analogy to the
natural one, is capable of destroying it; and this will be the
more easily effected in proportion as the symptoms of the
natural disease are prominent, characteristic, and decisive.

§ 179. But it more frequently happens that it is only in a
certain degree appropriate to the disease, and that it does not

suit exactly, because there was not a sufficient number of symptoms to direct the choice of the remedy.

§ 180. The medicine now operating upon a disease to which it is only partly analogous, excites accessory symptoms, as in the case (§ 162 and others) where the choice is imperfect, in consequence of the limited number of homœopathic remedies. It will then produce several appearances belonging to the mass of its own symptoms. *But these appearances are equally symptoms belonging to the disease itself, which the patient did not till now perceive, or he had rarely felt them,* and which now do nothing more than develop themselves in a greater degree.

§ 181. It will, perhaps, be objected that the accessory symptoms, or the new ones appearing in the disease, ought to be attributed to the remedy which had just been administered. This is indeed the source they spring from ;* but they are not less, on that account, symptoms that *this* disease itself was capable of producing in *this* patient, and the remedy in its character of exciting similar symptoms only provoked their manifestation. In short, the totality of the symptoms which then appear, ought to be regarded as belonging to the disease itself in its present state, and should be looked upon as such in the treatment.

* Unless they be occasioned by an important error of regimen, inflamed passions, or an impetuous movement in the organism, such as the establishment or cessation of the menses, conception, child-birth, &c.

§ 182. It is thus that the choice of the remedy (which must almost inevitably be imperfect, by reason of the few symptoms that show themselves) performs the office of perfecting the *ensemble* of the symptoms, and facilitates in this manner the discovery of a second and more appropriate homœopathic remedy.

§ 183. Unless the recently developed symptoms should be so violent as to call for immediate assistance, (which is rarely the case, on account of the minuteness of the homœopathic doses, especially in chronic diseases,) it is necessary, when the first remedy has produced no favourable results, to write down again the existing state of the disease, and select a second homœopathic remedy that is exactly suitable. This will be the easier performed in proportion as the group of symptoms is grown more numerous and complete.*

* A case that is very rare in chronic diseases, but which is sometimes met with in acute ones, is that where, notwithstanding the indistinctness of symptoms, the patient feels himself very ill, which may be ascribed to the depressed state of the sensibility that does not permit him to have a clear conception of the sufferings and symptoms. In a case of this nature, opium (in a high potence) will remove the torpor of the nervous system, and then the symptoms of the disease develop themselves plainly in the re-action of the organism.

§ 184. A similar course is to be continued after the full effects of each dose, and the state of disease that remains behind is to be noted down, describing the existing symptoms, and the image that results therefrom will serve to find a new remedy as homœopathic as possible. This method must be pursued until the cure is accomplished.

The treatment of diseases with local symptoms; their cure by means of external applications is always injurious.

§ 185. Among partial diseases, those which are called *local* hold a most important rank. By these, are meant the changes and sufferings experienced by the external part of the body. Until the present time, it has been the theory of the former schools of medicine that the external parts only were affected in such a case, and that the rest of the body did not participate in the disease : an absurd theoretical proposition that has led to the most pernicious medical treatment.

§ 186. The so-called local diseases of recent origin arising only from external causes seem more than others to be entitled to this name. But the injury must then be very trifling, and is of no particular importance ; for if the evils which attack the body externally are of any importance, the entire system sympathizes, and fever declares itself, &c. The treatment of these maladies belongs to surgery, so far as it is necessary to bring mechanical aid to the suffering parts, in order to remove and annihilate mechanical obstacles to the cure, which can only be expected from the powers of the organism itself. Among these may be ranked, for example, the reduction of dislocations ; uniting wounds by bandages ; extracting foreign substances that have penetrated the living parts ; opening the cavity of the abdomen, either to remove a substance that is burdensome to the system, or to give vent to effusions and collections of liquids ; placing in opposition the extremities of a fractured bone, and consolidation of the fracture by means of an appropriate bandage, &c. But as, when the injuries occur, the entire organism *always* requires active *dynamic* aid to be placed in a condition to accomplish the cure—when, for instance, it is necessary to have recourse to internal remedies to extinguish violent fever, arising from a severe contusion, a laceration of the soft parts—viz. muscles, tendons, and blood-vessels—or when it is requisite to combat homœopathically the external pain caused by a burn or cautery, then commence the functions of the dynamic physician, and the aid of homœo-pathy becomes necessary.

§ 187. But it is very different with the changes and mala-dies which occur on the surface of the body, not originating from any external violence. or merely from the consequences of some slight external injury. These owe their source to an internal affection. It is, therefore, equally absurd and dan-gerous to regard these diseases as symptoms that are purely local, and to treat them exclusively, or nearly so, by topical applications, as if they were surgical cases, in which manner they have been treated till the present day.

§ 188. These maladies have been considered as purely local, and, consequently, received the appellation of such, because they were looked upon as affections that were in a manner attached to the extreme parts in which the organism took little or no share, as if it was ignorant of their existence.*

* One of the many pernicious blunders of the old school.

§ 189. The slightest reflection, however, will suffice to explain why an external malady (which has not been occa-sioned by an important external violence) cannot arise, con-tinue, or much less grow worse, without some internal cause, the co-operation of the whole system, the latter, consequently, being diseased. It could never manifest itself if the general state of health was not immediately concerned, or if all the sensitive and irritable parts of the body did not participate.

Its production would be impossible, if it did not result from some modification of the entire principle of life, so closely are the parts of the body connected with each other, and form so inseparable a whole in regard to feeling and action. No eruption of the lips nor whitlow can take place without some internal derangement having been previously and simultaneously effected.

§ 190. All medical treatment of external diseases, that have arisen almost without any violence being exercised on the exterior of the body, ought, consequently, to have for its object the annihilation and cure of the general malady under which the organism suffers, by internal remedies. There is no other safe mode of curing them radically.

§ 191. This is confirmed by experience, which shows us that every energetic internal remedy produces, immediately after it has been administered, important changes in the general state of the patient, and particularly in that of the. external parts that are affected, (which the ordinary school of medicine look upon as isolated,) even in the so-called local affections, when they are situated at the extremities of the body. And these changes are of the most salutary nature; they consist of the cure of the entire body, and remove, at the same time, the local evil without the necessity of applying any external remedy, provided the internal one that is directed against the whole malady has been well selected and is perfectly homœopathic.

§ 192. The best method of effecting this object is, on examining the actual case of disease, to take into consideration not only the exact character of the local affection, but, in addition to that, every other change that is perceptible in the state of the patient. All these symptoms ought to be reunited in one perfect image, to be able to select a suitable homœopathic remedy from among the medicines whose morbid symptoms are already known.

§ 193. This remedy administered alone internally, and of which a single dose will suffice, when the disease is of recent origin, cures simultaneously the general bodily disease and the local affection. Such an effect on the part of the remedy ought to prove to us that the local evil depends solely upon a malady of the entire body, and that it ought to be considered as an inseparable part of the whole, and one of the most considerable and prominent symptoms of the general disease.

§ 194. It is not proper, either in acute local affections of recent origin, or in those which have already existed a long time, to make any topical application whatever to the diseased part, not even a substance which would be homœopathic or specific, if taken internally, or to administer it simultaneously with the internal medicinal agent. For acute local affections, such as inflammation, erysipelas, &c., which have not been produced by external injuries violent in proportion to their intensity, but by dynamic or internal causes, generally yield in a very short time to remedies capable of exciting an internal and external state similar to the one that actually exists.* If the disease is not wholly removed—if, notwithstanding the regularity of the mode of life of the patient, there still remains some local or general trace of it which the vital power is not able to restore to the normal state—then the acute local affection was (what happens very frequently) the product of psora, which had till then been latent in the interior of the organism, and which is now on the point of manifesting itself in a form of a chronic disease.

* For example, aconite, rhus toxicod., belladonna, mercury, &c.

§ 195. To perform a radical cure in these cases, which are by no means rare, it is necessary, after a tolerable abatement of the acute state, to direct an appropriate antipsoric treatment against the symptoms which continue to exist, together with those which the patient had been subject to previously, (according to the instructions given in the work *on chronic diseases**). An antipsoric treatment is, besides, requisite in local chronic affections that are manifestly not venereal.

* The second edition of this work is about to be translated, and will be published immediately.—EDITOR.

§ 196. It might be supposed that these diseases would be cured more promptly, if the remedy known to be homœopathic to the totality of the symptoms was employed, not only internally, but likewise externally, and that a medicine applied to

13

the spot itself that is diseased, ought then to produce a more rapid change.

§ 197.   But this method should be rejected not only in local affections which depend upon the miasm of psora, but also in those especially which result from the miasms of syphilis or sycosis. *For the simultaneous application of a remedy inter-nally and externally, in a disease whose principal symptom is a permanent local evil,* brings one serious disadvantage with it— the external affection* usually disappears faster than the internal malady, which gives rise to an erroneous impression that the cure is complete, or at least it becomes difficult, and sometimes impossible, to judge whether the entire disease has been destroyed or not by the internal remedy.

* Recent psoric eruption, chancre, sycosis.

§ 198.   The same motive ought to make us reject the *mere local application* of remedies to the external symptoms of chronic miasmatic diseases.   For if we confine ourselves to the suppression of the local symptoms, an impenetrable ob-scurity is then spread over the treatment, which is necessary to the perfect re-establishment of health : the principal symp-tom of the local affection is removed, and there only remain the others which are much less important and certain, and which are often not sufficiently characterized to furnish a clear and perfect image of the disease.

§ 199.   If the remedy homœopathic to the disease was not yet discovered* when the local symptom was destroyed by cauterization, excision, or desiccatives, the case becomes still more embarrassing, on account of the uncertainty and incon-stancy of the symptoms that remain.   And this difficulty is inevitable, because the external symptom which would have been the best guide in the choice of a remedy, and have pointed out the proper time of using it internally, is removed from our observation.

.* As was the case before my time with regard to anti-sycosic and anti-psoric remedies.

§ 200.   If this symptom still existed, it might have led to the discovery of the homœopathic remedy suitable to the entire malady ; this remedy once discovered, the continued

existence of the local affection would show that the cure was
not yet perfected, while its disappearance would prove that the
evil had been extirpated to the very root, and the cure absolute, an advantage that cannot be too highly appreciated.

§ 201. It is evident that the vital power, charged with a
chronic disease which it cannot subdue by its own energy,
does not adopt the measure of exciting a local affection on
any external part whatever, but for the purpose of allaying
(by abandoning to its power those organs whose integrity is
not absolutely necessary to existence) an internal disease
which threatens to destroy the essential springs of life. Its
object is, in a manner, to transport the malady from one spot
to another, and substitute an external evil in the place of one
that is internal. In this way the local affection silences, for a
while, the internal malady, but without being able either to
cure or diminish it in a great degree.* The local malady,
however, is never anything more than a part of the general
disease, but it is a part that the vital power has (*einseitige*)
greatly magnified, and which she has carried back to the surface of the body where there is less danger, in order to diminish the internal affection in an equal degree. But this latter
is not the less cured on that account: on the contrary, it
makes a gradual progress, so that the organism is likewise
compelled to enlarge and aggravate the local symptom, in
order to replace it to a certain extent, and procure for it
partial relief. Thus, old ulcers in the legs grow large so long
as the internal psora is not cured, and chancres increase in
size as long as the internal syphilis remains without cure, just
as the internal disease of the whole body grows and enlarges
of itself.

* The issues of the old school produce something that is analogous.
These ulcers, created by art on the external parts, may, though for a very
short time, allay several internal chronic diseases, but they can never cure
them; on the other hand, they weaken and destroy the health far more than
the instinctive vital power does, by the most of its metastases.

§ 202. If the physician who has imbibed the precepts of the
ordinary school destroys the local malady by an external
remedy, thinking by these means to cure the disease itself, nature replaces this affection by increasing the internal suffer-

ings, and rousing all the other symptoms that already existed
with the local malady, and which appear to have been till that
time in a latent state. It is, therefore, erroneous that the external remedies have (as usually asserted) then driven back
the local malady into the body, or that they have thrown it
upon the nerves.

§ 203.   Every external treatment of a local symptom whose
aim is to extinguish it on the surface of the body without curing the internal miasmatic disease—such, for example, as that
of destroying a psoric eruption on the skin by means of ointments, healing up a chancre by the use of caustic, destroying
the granulations of sycosis by ligature, excision, or the application of a hot iron—is not only useless but injurious.   This
pernicious method, in such general use at the present day, is
the chief source of the innumerable chronic diseases (with or
without names) that oppress the human race.   This is the
most criminal practice physicians can adopt, and it has notwithstanding been very generally practised till the present
time, and taught, *ex cathedra*, as the only one.*

* For all the medicines which are directed to be given inwardly during
the local treatment, serve only to aggravate the evil, since they possess no
specific power to remove the entire disease, but assault and weaken the organism, and, in addition, inflict on it other chronic medicinal diseases.

*All diseases properly chronic, and not arising or being supported merely by
bad modes of living, ought to be treated by homœopathic remedies appropriate to their originating miasm, and solely by the internal administration
of those remedies.*

§ 204.   If we except all chronic maladies which depend
upon a mode of living habitually unhealthy, as well as those
innumerable factitious diseases (v. § 74) which arise from the
senseless and protracted, the assaulting and ruinous treatment,
even of slight diseases, by allœopathic physicians, then all the
remainder, without exception, are occasioned by the development of these three chronic miasms, viz., internal syphilis,
internal sycosis, but especially, and in an infinitely greater
proportion, internal psora.   Each of these is already in possession of the entire organism, and has penetrated it in all
its parts, before the respective primary representative and
local symptom makes its appearance, which prevents the
bursting forth of its corresponding miasm in another form, and

is manifested in psora by a peculiar eruption, in syphilis by chancre or bubo, and in sycosis by condylomata. Either of these chronic miasms being deprived of its local symptoms, will, sooner or later, under the influence of natural causes, become developed, burst forth, and multiply the incredible multitude of chronic diseases which for ages has afflicted the human race. These diseases never would have existed in such abundance, had physicians strenuously endeavoured to effect a radical cure of these three miasms, and to extinguish them from the organism, by means of the internal employment of homœopathic remedies adapted to each, without treating the external symptoms by topical applications.

§ 205. The homœopathic physician never treats the primitive symptoms of chronic miasms, nor the secondary evils that result from their development, by local remedies acting in a dynamic[1] or mechanical manner. But as this was not the method adopted by his predecessors, and as he generally finds the primitive symptoms[2] already effaced from the exterior, he has, for the most part, to treat secondary symptoms, evils provoked by the development of these inherent miasms, and more frequently chronic diseases that are the results of internal psora. On this head, I refer the reader to my treatise on chronic diseases, in which I have pointed out the system that is to be pursued in as precise a manner as it was possible for a single individual to do, after many years of experience, observation and reflection.

[1] Consequently, I cannot, for example, advise the local destruction of cancer in the lip or face (the result of psora strongly developed?) by the arsenical ointment of *frère Côme*; not only because this treatment is extremely painful, and frequently fails, but more particularly because such a dynamic remedy, although it may locally cleanse the body of the cancerous ulcer, does not in the slightest degree diminish the psora, which is the original disease, so that the preservative vital power is forced to carry back the focus of the great internal disease upon a more essential part, (as it happens in every case of metastasis,) and thus occasions blindness, deafness, madness, suffocative asthma, dropsy, apoplexy, &c. But arsenic ointment does not even reach so far as to destroy the local ulceration, except where the latter is of no very great extent, and the vital power retains great energy; but even in such a state of things, it is still possible to cure the original disease completely. The extirpation of cancer in the face or breast. or that of an encysted tumour, absolutely produces the same result. The operation is followed by a state

still more grievous, or at least the life of the patient is shortened. This in innumerable instances has been the result ; but still the old school, in its blindness, continues to produce in every new case the same calamity.

 ² Psoric eruption, chancre, (bubones,) sycosis.

Preliminary search after the simple miasm which forms the basis of the malady, or of its complication with a second (sometimes even with a third.)

§ 206. Previous to commencing the cure of a chronic disease, it is necessary to inquire with the greatest care* whether the patient has been affected with the venereal disease (or gonorrhea sycosica) ; for where this is the case, the treatment ought to be specially and solely directed towards these objects when no other symptoms but those of syphilis or sycosis are present, a circumstance that very rarely occurs in modern times. It is equally requisite, in the cure of internal psora, to inquire if an infection of this nature has taken place, because in that case there is a complication of those two diseases, as there always is when the symptoms of psora are not pure. Generally, when the physician thinks he has an old case of venereal disease before him, it is chiefly a complication of syphilis and psora that offers itself to his view, the internal psora being the *most frequent fundamental cause of chronic diseases,* whatever names they may bear, and which, by alloeopathic unskilfulness, has been, in addition, frequently marred and enormously heightened and disfigured.

* In making inquiries of this nature, the physician must not allow himself to be imposed on either by the assertions of the patients or those of their parents, who, even in the most inveterate cases of chronic diseases, assign for their cause a cold caught many years previous, a former fright, grief, witchcraft, &c. These causes are much too slight to produce a chronic disease in a healthy body, or to keep it up for a period of long duration, and render it worse from year to year, as is the case with all chronic diseases arising from the development of psora. Far more important causes than these must have presided at the birth of a severe chronic disease, and those which have just been enumerated could do nothing more than call forth a chronic miasm from its state of lethargy.

Inquiries to be made respecting the treatment previously adopted.

§ 207. The preceding examination being accomplished, then it is requisite for the homoeopathic physician to inquire what was the alloeopathic treatment adopted during the chronic disease—what powerful medicines especially and frequently were employed, the mineral waters used, and their effects. This information is necessary, in order that he may conceive, in some degree, the deviation from the primitive state, and, if possible, partially correct these artificial changes, or, at all events, that he may avoid the medicines already misapplied.

Other inquiries necessary to be made, before a perfect image can be formed of a chronic disease.

§ 208. The next step is to learn the age of the patient, his mode of life, regimen, occupation, domestic situation, social connections, &c. He is to examine whether these various circumstances contribute to increase the disease, and to what extent they may be favourable or unfavourable to the treatment. He must likewise endeavour to learn whether the patient's state of mind is any obstacle to the cure, and whether it be necessary to modify, favour, or direct it.

§ 209. It is not till after repeated inquiries of this nature that the physician should endeavour to trace out, according to the directions already given, as perfect an image of the disease as possible, to enable him to distinguish the most prominent and characteristic of the symptoms by which he is to choose the first antipsoric or other remedy, at the commencement of the treatment, observing as a guide, the greatest possible analogy with the symptoms, &c.

Treatment of mental diseases.

§ 210. Almost all those which I before designated by the name of partial (*einseitige*) diseases belong to psora, and seem on that account, more difficult to cure, because all their other symptoms disappear before that one great prevailing symptom. To these belong the so-called *diseases of the mind and temper.* These affections, however, do not form a distinct and wholly separate class from the others, for the state of the mind and temper varies in all other so-called bodily diseases,* and it ought to be comprised as one of the principal symptoms, of which it is important to note the whole, in order to trace a faithful image of the disease, and to be able to combat it with success, homœopathically.

§ 211. This extends so far that the moral state of the
patient is often that which is most decisive in the choice of
the homœopathic remedy; for this is a symptom of the most
precise character, and one that, among the mass of symptoms,
by no means can escape the notice of a physician accustomed
to make precise observations.

§ 212. The creator of medicinal agents has also been sin-
gularly attentive to this principal element of all diseases—the
changes in the state of mind and disposition: for there is not a
single operative medicine that does not effect a notable change
in the temper and manner of thinking of a healthy individual
to whom it is administered, and each medicinal substance
produces a different modification.

§ 213. No cure, then, can ever be performed according to
nature—that is to say, in a homœopathic manner—without
paying attention, at the same time, in every disease, and even
in those which are acute, to the change that has taken place
in the mind and disposition, and selecting a remedy capable
in itself of producing not only similar symptoms to those of
the malady, but also a similar disposition and state of mind.*

* Aconite seldom or ever effects a rapid and permanent cure when the
temper of the patient is quiet and even; or the nux-vomica, when the disposition is mild and phlegmatic; or pulsatilla, when it is lively, serene, or obstinate; or ignatia, when the mind is unchangeable and little susceptible of
either fear or grief.

§ 214. What I have to say regarding the treatment of
mental diseases may be comprised in a few words, for they

cannot be cured in a different manner from other diseases—
that is to say, it is necessary to oppose to them a remedy possessing a morbific power as similar as possible to the disease
itself in the effect which it produces upon the mind and body
of persons in health.

§ 215. Almost all affections of the mind and disposition
are nothing more than diseases of the body, in which the
changes of the moral faculties are (more or less rapidly) become predominant over all the other symptoms, which are diminished ; they finish by assuming the character of a partial
disease and almost of a local affection.

§ 216. In the so-called bodily diseases which are dangerous, such as suppuration of the lungs, or that of any other
essential viscera, or another acute disease, viz., in childbed,
&c., where the intensity of the moral symptom increases
rapidly, the disease turns to insanity, melancholy, or madness,
which removes the danger arising from the bodily symptoms.
The latter improve so far as almost to be restored to a healthy
state, or rather they are diminished in such a degree as to be
no longer perceptible but to the eye of the observer gifted
with penetration and perseverance. In this manner they
degenerate into a partial (*einseitige*) disease, even as if local,
in which the moral symptom, very slight in the first instance,
assumes so great a preponderance that it becomes the most
prominent of all—substitutes itself in a great degree for the
others, and subdues their virulence by acting on them as a
palliative. In short, the disease of the bodily organs, which
are grosser in their nature, has been transported to the almost
spiritual organs of the mind, which no anatomist ever could
or will be able to reach with his scalpel.

§ 217. In affections of this kind, it is requisite to proceed
with particular care in searching for the entire signs both in
regard to the bodily symptoms and more especially that of the
principal and characteristic symptom—the state of the mind
and disposition. By these means alone can we succeed in discovering, among the number of medicines whose pure effects
are known, a remedy that has the power of extinguishing the
entire evil at once ; for it is necessary that, among the num-

ber of the symptoms peculiar to this remedy, there should be some which resemble as closely as possible not only the bodily symptoms of the disease, but also its moral ones in particular.

§ 218.   To obtain possession of this totality of the symptoms, it is requisite, in the first place, to describe with precision all those which the disease exhibited previous to the moment when, by the preponderance of the moral symptoms, it changed to an affection of the mind and disposition.   This information will be furnished by the persons who are about the patient.

§ 219.   By comparing these previous symptoms of the bodily disease with the traces of those that still remain, but which are nearly effaced, (and perceptible at lucid intervals, or when the mental affection undergoes a transitory diminution,) we may satisfy ourselves that although they were concealed, still they never ceased to exist.

§ 220.   If we add to all this, the state of mind and disposition which the persons around the patient, and the physician himself, has observed with the greatest care, we have then arrived at the perfect image of the malady, and may proceed to look for the homœopathic remedy that is to cure it—that is to say, (if the mental affection has already existed a long time,) for the anti-psoric remedy, which has the power of exciting similar symptoms, and principally an analogous disorder in the moral faculties.

§ 221.   If, however, the ordinary calm and tranquil state of the patient has been suddenly changed by the influence of fear, grief, spirituous liquors, &c., to one of madness or furor, thus presenting the character of an acute disease, although the affection is almost always the result of internal psora, like a raging flame bursting forth from it, yet the physician cannot attempt to combat it immediately by the use of antipsoric remedies.   It is necessary first to oppose to it other medicines —such, for example, as aconite, belladonna, stramonium, hyosciamus, mercury, &c., in highly developed, minute doses—in order to allay it sufficiently to bring back the psora to its former latent condition, which gives the patient the appearance of being cured.

§ 222.   But a patient who has thus been freed from an

acute disease of the mind or disposition by the use of non-anti-psoric remedies, can never be regarded as cured. Far from it; and it is necessary to lose no time in placing him under a prolonged antipsoric treatment to deliver him of the chronic miasm of psora, which, it is true, has again become latent, but is not less ready on that account to break out again.* In short, there is no fear of another attack similar to that which has been arrested, provided the patient does not depart from the regimen that has been prescribed for him.

* It is a very rare case that mental alienation of long standing ceases spontaneously, (since the internal malady recedes upon the grosser corporeal organs.) These are the few cases in which a patient, after having been the inmate of a mad-house, is discharged as apparently cured. Every institution for the insane has hitherto been filled to excess, so that the multitude of others waiting for admission have scarcely ever found a place, if vacancies did not occur in the house by the decease of patients. *Not one among them is really and permanently cured!* A striking evidence this, among many others, of the complete nullity of the pernicious treatment hitherto pursued, which allœopathic ostentation has ridiculously honoured with the title of the rational art of healing. On the other hand, how often have these unfortunate beings, by means of a treatment purely homœopathic, been restored to the possession of their mental and bodily health, and returned to their gratified connections and the world !

§ 223. But where the antipsoric treatment is discontinued, it is almost certain that a much slighter cause than that which excited the first appearance of insanity will suffice to bring on a fresh and more permanent attack of it, during which psora develops itself in a perfect manner, and it will then turn to a periodical or permanent mental alienation, which can with difficulty be cured by antipsorics.

§ 224. In a case where the mental disease is not yet completely formed, and where it is doubtful whether it really results from bodily affection, or if it is not rather the effects of bad education, evil habits, corrupted morals, a neglected mind, superstition, or ignorance, the truth will be readily discovered by acting as follows. The patient is to be addressed in a tone of friendly exhortation, while motives of consolation, serious remonstrances, and solid arguments, are to be urged on the occasion: if the disorder of the mind does not proceed from a bodily disease, it will readily yield to such means; but if the contrary is the case, the malady rapidly grows worse, the melancholic becomes still more grave, downcast, and inconsolable, the wicked maniac more outrageous, and the unmeaning prattler more foolish.*

* It seems as though the mind were sensible of the truth of these representations, and acted upon the body as if it would restore the lost harmony, but that the latter reacts, by means of a disease, upon the organs of the mind and disposition, and augments the derangement which already exists, by throwing back on them its own peculiar sufferings.

§ 225. But, as we have just witnessed, there are likewise a few mental diseases that do not owe their origin solely to a bodily disease, but which, on the contrary, with a slight indisposition, have been produced by moral affections, such as continued grief, anger, injured feelings, or great and repeated occasions of fear and alarm. In the course of time, these latter have an influence over the health of the body, and often compromise it in a high degree.

§ 226. It is merely in mental diseases, thus engendered and kept up by the disposition itself, that moral remedies are to be relied on, and that only *while they are still recent, and have not yet made any great inroad upon the physical state of the organism.* In this case, it is possible that treating the patient with a show of confidence, bestowing on him friendly exhortations and sensible advice, and sometimes practising on him a deception that is disguised with art, will soon restore the health of the mind, and then, with the aid of a suitable regimen, the body also may apparently be brought back to its normal condition.

§ 227. But these maladies are likewise the results of a psoric miasm that was not yet ready to devolop itself in a perfect manner, and prudence requires that the patient should be submitted to a radical antipsoric cure, to prevent a relapse (which too often occurs) of the same mental affection.

§ 228. In mental diseases that are produced by an affection of the body, whose cure can alone be effected by a homœopathic antipsoric remedy, aided by a careful and regular mode of life, it is also proper to join to this treatment a certain regimen for the government of the mind. In this respect it is necessary that the physician, and those about the patient, should scrupulously observe that line of conduct towards him that has been judged suitable. To the furious maniac, we are to oppose tranquillity and unshaken firmness, free from fear; to the patient who vents his sufferings in grief and lamentation, silent pity that is expressed by the countenance and gestures; to senseless prattle, a silence not wholly inattentive; to disgusting and detestable demeanour and similar discourse, entire inattention. What regards the injury and damage that a maniac may commit, we are only to anticipate and prevent it without ever expressing a word of reproach to him; everything ought to be so ordered, that punishments and the infliction of bodily sufferings may be dispensed with.* And this can be effected without any great difficulty, since in administering the medicine (the only point where the use of coercive measures would be justifiable) the dose in the homœopathic treatment is so small that the medicinal substance never offends the taste, and the patient can be made to swallow it in his drink without ever perceiving it.

* It is surprising to witness the hard-hearted and imprudent treatment adopted in several mad-houses, not only in England, but also in Germany, by physicians who, ignorant of the only true method of curing mental disease by the aid of homœopathic (antipsoric) remedies, do nothing more than beat and torture the unfortunate beings who are so worthy of compassion. By this revolting mode of treatment, they lower themselves beneath the rank of the common jailer in the houses of correction; for it is in virtue of his office, and upon criminals only, that the latter exercises his cruelty, while the physician, either too ignorant or indolent to go in search of a suitable method in treatment, only appears to exert his tyranny upon the innocent patient through spite, because he is not able to cure him.

§ 229. On the other hand, contradiction, zealous remonstrance, violence, and reproaches, are as inapplicable and injurious in the treatment of mental disease as are indecision and timidity. But mockery, in particular, and deception, which the maniac is not slow in perceiving, only irritate and provoke him. *The physician, and those who guard the patient, ought always to appear as if they believed him to be possessed of reason.* It is likewise necessary to remove from his view all external objects that could disturb or afflict him. There is no relief or distraction for the clouded mind—no salutary recreation—no means of instruction or consolation either in books, conversation, or otherwise, for the soul that languishes in the prison of a diseased body—nothing can procure him repose but the cure of his bodily sufferings, and he is equally a stranger to comfort and tranquillity until reason is restored.

§ 230. If the antipsoric remedy that is to be used in any given case of mental affection, of which there are an endless variety of cases, be perfectly homœopathic to the true image of the disease, (which is easily discovered when the number of known medicines is sufficiently great that the principal symptom, viz., the moral state of the patient, is strongly developed,) then the smaller dose often suffices to produce, in a short time, a very decided amelioration, which could not have been obtained by all the other (allœopathic) remedies administered in large doses, and lavished on the patient till he was near death. I can even affirm, after long experience, that the superiority of homœopathy over every other curative method whatever, was never more manifest than in mental diseases of long standing, which owed their origin to bodily affections, or which were developed simultaneously.

Intermittent and alternating diseases.

§ 231. There is yet another class of diseases that merits our particular attention. These are the intermittent diseases, such as return at stated periods like the innumerable intermittent fevers, and the non-febrile affections assuming the same form, and also those which in certain morbid states alternate with others at indefinite intervals.

§ 232. These latter (*alternating*) species are likewise in great variety;* but they all belong to the number of chronic diseases. The greater part of them result from a development of psora, sometimes, but rarely, complicated with a syphilitic miasm. This is the reason that they are cured in the first instance by antipsoric medicines, and in the second by antipsorics, alternating with anti-syphilitics, as I have stated in my Treatise on Chronic Diseases.

* It is possible for two or three different states to alternate with each other. For example, in a case that regards the alternation of two different states, it can happen that certain pains may be produced in the lower extremities as soon as ophthalmia disappears, and the latter may return again

immediately when the pains have ceased—or that spasms and convulsions may immediately succeed some other affection, either of the entire body or one of its parts. But it is also possible, in the case of a triple alliance of alternative states in a quotidian complaint, that an apparent superabundance of health, an exaltation of the faculties of the mind and body, (such as unusual gaiety, excessive vivacity. an exaggerated feeling of comfort, immoderate appetite, &c.) may be abruptly succeeded by a downcast and melancholy humour, an insupportable tendency to hypochondriasis, and a derangement of several of the vital functions (digestion, sleep, &a.) : and this second may make room in a less sudden manner to the feeling of indisposition which the patient was subject to in ordinary times. Sometimes there is no longer any trace whatever of the anterior state when the new one has established itself. Sometimes there are vestiges of it still remaining. In certain cases, the morbid states that succeed each other and in their nature directly opposite —as, for example, melancholy and mirthful insanity, or furor, alternating periodically.

Typical intermittent diseases.

§ 233. The *typical intermittents* are those wherein a morbid state, resembling that which previously existed, re-appears at the expiration of a certain interval of apparent recovery, and vanishes again after having lasted for an equal period of time. This phenomenon not only occurs in the great variety of intermittent fevers, but likewise in diseases that are apparently without fever, which appear and disappear at regular periods.

§ 234. Those morbid states, apparently without fever, which assume a particular type—that is to say, which return at fixed periods in the same patient (they do not manifest themselves, in general, either sporadically or epidemically)—all belong to the class of chronic diseases. The greater number of them depend on a simple psoric affection, seldom complicated with syphilis, and they are combated successfully by the same treatment. It is, however, sometimes necessary to have recourse to a very small dose of extenuated solution of cinchona, for the purpose of completely extinguishing their intermittent form.

Intermittent fevers.

§ 235. With respect to *intermittent fevers** that manifest themselves sporadically or epidemically, (not the endemics of marshy districts,) we often find that each of their attacks or paroxysms is likewise composed of two contrary morbid states

of cold and heat, or heat and cold ; but most frequently it consists of three—cold, heat, and perspiration. For this reason
it is, therefore, necessary that the remedy employed against
them, which is to be selected from the medicines hitherto tried,
commonly from the non-antipsorics, shall likewise (as the
surest means) be able to excite in healthy persons two (or all
three) of the morbid stages that are similar; or, at least, it shall
have the faculty of exciting, with all its accessory symptoms,
the strongest and most prominent of these two or three consecutive stages, viz., either that of chill, with its accessory
symptoms, or of heat, with the symptoms accompanying it, or
of perspiration, with its attendant complaints, according as the
one or the other stage may be the strongest and most distinguished; yet the state of the patient, during the apyrexia,
especially, must indicate the choice of the most appropriate
homœopathic remedy.

* Till the present time, pathology has only been acquainted with one single
intermittent fever, which has been called *ague*. It admits of no other difference than the interval which exists between the paroxysms ; and upon this
are founded the particular denominations, quotidian, tertian, quartan, &c. But,
besides the variety which they present in regard to the periods of their return,
the intermittent fevers exhibit yet other changes that are much more important. Among these fevers there are many which cannot be denominated
ague, because, their attacks consist solely of heat ; others are characterized
by cold only, succeeded or not by perspiration ; while yet others freeze the
body of the patient, and inspire him, notwithstanding, with a sensation of heat,
or even create in him a feeling of cold, although his body seems very warm
to the touch ; in many, one of the paroxysms is confined to shivering or cold,
which is immediately succeeded by a comfortable sensation, and that which
comes after it consists of heat followed by perspiration or not. In one case,
it is heat that manifests itself first, and cold succeeds ; in another, both the
cold and heat give place to apyrexia, while the next paroxysm, which sometimes does not occur before an interval of several hours, consists merely of
perspiration ; in certain cases, no trace of perspiration is perceptible ; while
in others the attack is composed solely of perspiration, without either heat or
cold, or of perspiration that flows during the heat alone. There exist, likewise, innumerable differences relative to the accessory symptoms, the particular kind of headache, the bad taste in the mouth, the stomach sickness,
the vomiting, the diarrhœa, the absence or degree of thirst, the kind of pains
felt in the body and limbs, sleep, delirium, changes of the temper, spasms,
&c., which manifest themselves before, during, or after the cold, hot, or
sweating stages, without taking into the account a multitude of other deviations. These are assuredly intermittent fevers that are very different from

one another, each of which demands naturally that mode of homœopathic treatment that is appropriate to it individually. It must be confessed, it is true, that they may almost all be suppressed (a case that so frequently occurs) by large and enormous doses of cinchona or quinine—that is to say, cinchona prevents their periodical return, and destroys the type. But when this remedy is employed in intermittent fevers where it is inappropriate, (as is the case with all epidemic intermittents which pass over whole countries, and even mountains,) the patient is not at all cured, because the character of the disease is destroyed; he is still indisposed, and often much more so than he was before; he suffers from a peculiar chronic bark complaint, often incurable, and yet this is what physicians term a cure.

§ 236. The best, most appropriate, and serviceable method in these diseases, is to administer the remedy immediately, or very shortly after the termination of the paroxysm, as soon as the patient has, in some measure, recovered from it. Administered in this manner, it has sufficient time to produce in the organism all its various effects to restore health without violence or commotion; whereas, if taken immediately before the paroxysm, (even though it were homœopathic or specific in the highest degree,) its effect would coincide with the renewal of the natural disease, and excite such a strife in the organism, so powerful a reaction, that the patient would lose at least a great portion of his strength, and even life would be endangered.* But when the medicine is administered immediately after the termination of the paroxysm, and before the next fit has prepared itself, even at a distance, to appear, the organism is in the best possible condition to allow itself to be gently modified by the remedy, and by these means return to a state of health.

* There are proofs of this, unfortunately, in the too frequent cases where a moderate allœopathic dose of opium, administered to the patient during the cold stage of the fever, has quickly deprived him of life.

§ 237. If the period of the apyrexia be of short duration, as is the case in some very violent fevers, or if it be disturbed by symptoms which belong to the preceding paroxysm, then it is necessary to administer the homœopathic remedy as soon as the perspiration or other symptoms, pointing out the termination of the fit, begin to diminish.

§ 238. When a single dose of the appropriate remedy has destroyed several paroxysms, and manifestly restored health,

and, notwithstanding which, indications of a fresh attack are
seen some time after, then only can and ought the same remedy to be repeated, provided the totality of the symptoms is
still the same. But this return of the same fever, after an
interval of health, is not possible, except when the cause
which excited the malady, in the first instance, still exercises
its influence upon the convalescent, as occurs in marshy countries. In such a case, a permanent cure is seldom effected but
by removing the patient from this exciting cause, and advising
him to go and reside in a mountainous district, if that which
attacked him was a marsh intermittent fever.

§ 239. As almost every medicine, in its simple action, produces a peculiar fever, and even a species of intermittent,
which differs from all those excited by other medicines, consequently the immense number of medicinal substances presents
the means of combating all natural intermittent fevers homœopathically. Some efficacious remedies against a multitude of
these affections, have already been discovered in a few medicines that have been tried, till the present time, on healthy
individuals.

§ 240. When a remedy is found to be homœopathic or
specific in a reigning epidemy of intermittent fevers, and there
is, notwithstanding, now and then, a patient whom it does not
cure in a perfect manner, and no influence of a marshy
country opposes its operation, then the obstacle generally
arises from the psoric miasm, and, consequently, antipsoric
medicines ought to be employed until health is perfectly
restored.

§ 241. Epidemical intermittent fevers, in places where
none are endemic, have the nature of chronic diseases, composed of individual, acute paroxysms. Each particular epidemic has a peculiar character, *per se*, that is shared in
common by every patient affected by it, and which, when it is
discovered in the totality of symptoms common to all, indicates the suitable homœopathic remedy (specific) for all the
cases; and this remedy is almost universally effectual in
patients who had enjoyed tolerable health before the onset of
the epidemic, that is, who suffered under no chronic malady
from developed psora.

§ 242. If, however, in such an epidemic intermittent, the first paroxysms have passed over uncured, or if the patient's strength had been reduced by improper allœopathic treatment, then the internal psoric miasm (though slumbering, yet unfortunately existing in so many persons) develops itself, assumes here the intermittent type, and, in appearance, continues to play the part of the intermittent fever itself, so that the medicine (rarely an antipsoric) which would have been beneficial in the incipient paroxysms, is now no longer suitable or capable of affording relief. The disease at present to be combated has generated into a psoric intermittent, which is generally overcome by means of a minute dose, seldom repeated, of sulphur and sulphuretum calcis, of the highest developments.

§ 243. Those frequently very malignant intermittent fevers which attack an individual here and there, not inhabiting marshy regions, must, in the commencement, be treated as acute diseases, (to which they bear some resemblance, as regards their psoric origin,) by selecting a homœopathic remedy, for the special case, from the class of the other proven (non-antipsoric) medicines, which is to be continued for some days with the view of affording the greatest possible relief. But if the recovery should be lingering, it must be seen that psora is now on the point of development, and that a radical cure cannot be effected without antipsoric remedies.

§ 244. The endemic intermittent fevers of marshy districts and countries subject to inundations are a source of much embarrassment to physicians of the prevailing school of medicine. A healthy man may, however, accustom himself in his youth to the influence of a country that is covered with morasses, and live there in perfect health, provided he confines himself to a regular mode of life, and is not assailed by want, fatigue, or destructive passions. The endemic intermittent fevers will at farthest attack him on his first arrival in the country : but one or two of the smallest doses of a solution of cinchona, attenuated in a very high degree, suffice to deliver him from it promptly, if, in other respects, he does not depart from a strict regimen. But when a man, who takes sufficient bodily exercise, and who pursues a course every way suited to his mind

and body, does not cure of a marsh intermittent fever by the
influence of this single remedy, we may be certain that there
exists within his body a psoric affection, which is on the eve
of developing itself, and that the intermittent fever will not
yield to any other than an antipsoric treatment.* It sometimes happens, that if this man quit the marshy country without delay, to go and reside in another that is dry and mountainous, his health is apparently restored, and the fever leaves
him, if it has not taken too deep a root—that is to say, the
psora passes again to a latent state, because it had not yet
reached its final degree of development ; but he is not cured,
nor can he enjoy perfect health, until he has made use of an
antipsoric treatment.

* Large doses of cinchona or sulphate of quinine may certainly free the
patient from the typical attacks of marsh intermittent fevers ; but he is still
unhealthy in another way, and antipsorics only will effect a perfect cure.

The mode of administering the remedies.

§ 245. Having now seen what degree of attention ought,
in the homœopathic treatment, to be bestowed on the principal diversities of diseases and their peculiar circumstances,
we pass on to the *remedies themselves, the manner of applying
them, and the regimen to be observed* by the patient during the
time he is submitted to their action. Both in acute and
chronic diseases, every perceptible amelioration that takes
place making continual progress, though of ever so feeble a
nature, is a state which, as long as it endures, formally for-
bids the repetition of any medicine whatever, because the one
already taken by the patient has not yet produced all the
good that may result from it. Every fresh dose of a remedy,
even of the one last administered, and which had till then
proved salutary, would have no effect but that of disturbing
the operation of the cure.

§ 246. On the contrary, one dose of a suitable homœopathic remedy, if its development be sufficiently subtile, gradually completes all the beneficial effects which, from its nature,
it is capable of producing, and provided its operation be undisturbed, sometimes in the space of forty, fifty, to one hundred days. This, however, is seldom the case ; and it depends

upon the physician as well as upon the patient, whether these periods may not be abridged to the extent of one-half, one-fourth, or even to a shorter time, and thus a more speedy cure effected. Recent and abundant experience has taught us that this may be happily accomplished under three conditions: first, when a remedy has been chosen with due circumspection—that is, strikingly homœopathic; secondly, when it is administered in the highest development, the least revolting to the vital power, and yet sufficiently energetic to influence it; and thirdly, when such a subtile, energetic dose of the best-selected remedy *is repeated at the most suitable intervals*,* which experience has determined for accelerating the cure, yet, in fulfilling this condition, it is requisite that the vital power to be influenced to the production of the similar medicinal disease, may not be excited to disagreeable counteraction.

* In the former editions of the Organon I have recommended that a single dose of a well-chosen homœopathic remedy be permitted to complete its operation, before a repetition of the same, or an administration of another remedy—a doctrine which was the result of certain experience, it being ascertained that too large a dose even of a well-selected remedy, (which, as if by a retrograde course, has been of late again proposed,) or what is the same thing, numerous small doses, repeated in quick succession, rarely ever effected the greatest possible benefit in the cure of diseases, and particularly of the chronic. Because, by such a practice, the vital power, in its transition from the state induced by natural disease to that of a similar medicinal one, cannot tranquilly adapt itself to the change, but generally becomes so violently excited from a large dose, or the frequent repetition of smaller doses even of a homœopathic remedy, that, in most cases, its reaction is anything rather than salutary; in short, it is more injurious than useful. As long as nothing more beneficial was at that time discovered, than the practice then taught by me, the philanthropic precautionary rule, *si non juvat, modo ne noceat*, enjoined upon the homœopathic physician who regarded the good of his species as his highest aim, to administer in diseases, generally, but one and the smallest dose of the suitable remedy, and to wait for its complete effect. I say the smallest dose, since it will stand good as a homœopathic rule of cure, refutable by no experience whatever, that the best dose of the rightly-selected medicine is ever the smallest, and in one of the higher developments (X°) for chronic as well as acute diseases—a truth which is the invaluable property of pure homœopathy, and which, so long as allœopathy (and what is but little short of it, the practice of the new mongrel sect, consisting in a combination of allœopathy and homœopathy) continues to gnaw like a cancer upon the vitals of diseased beings, and to destroy them with large doses of medicine, will separate these pretended arts by an immeasurable gulf from homœopathy.

On the other hand, although practice points out to us that a single small dose is sufficient in some cases of disease, particularly those of a lighter kind, and in those of small children and adults of a tender and irritable constitution, to produce almost all that the medicine is capable of producing, yet in most cases, both of chronic disease of long standing, (often previously almost ruined by the use of improper medicines,) as well as in important acute diseases, such a minute dose, even when given in the higher developments, is manifestly not sufficient to perform all the curative effects which was to have been expected from one and the same medicine. For this purpose, unquestionably, it becomes necessary to administer several of the same, and thereby the vital power may be pathogenetically influenced, and its healthy reaction extended so high, that it may wholly obliterate all that portion of the original disease which the well-selected homœopathic remedy is capable of doing. One small dose of the best selected medicine produces, indeed, some relief, but not sufficient.

But the careful homœopathic physician will not venture frequently to repeat a dose of the same remedy, at short intervals, because no advantage is derived from this practice, but more frequently, as is attested by accurate observation, it is the source of certain injury. He generally sees an aggravation of the symptoms, even from the smallest dose of a suitable remedy, which, on being given to-day, is repeated to-morrow and the day following.

In order to afford greater relief in cases where he is convinced that the remedy is the most fitly chosen, than has been hitherto effected by prescribing only one small dose, it naturally occurred to the physician to enlarge it, (since, for the reasons aforementioned, it was to be administered once only,) and instead of one minute globule moistened with the medicine in the highest development, to give six or eight at once, or even a whole or half a drop. But, almost without exception, the results of this practice were less favourable than they ought to have been, often really injurious and of difficult reparation.

Neither did the substitution of the lower dilutions administered in larger doses furnish any better expedient.

To increase the strength of the dose of a homœopathic remedy sufficient for producing the supposed degree of pathogenetic excitement of the vital powers requisite for salutary and sufficient reaction, fulfils, therefore, as experience teaches, by no means the desired intention. The vital power is thereby too violently and too suddenly assaulted to allow of time for a gradual, equable, and salutary counteraction; in order to accommodate itself to its change, therefore, it endeavours to rid itself, as if of an enemy, of the medicinal influence, pressed upon it in excess, by means of vomiting, diarrhœa, sweat, fever, &c., and thus, in great measure, frustrates the aim of the indiscreet physician. By this practice, little or nothing is effected in the cure of the disease, rather is the patient thereby debilitated, and a long time must elapse before the smallest dose of the same remedy can be repeated, if it shall not operate injuriously.

But a number of small doses given in rapid succession with the same view, accumulate in the system, and form, collectively, an excessive dose, (a few rare cases excepted,) with similar evil consequences. In this case, the vital power, being unable to recover itself in the interval between the repetition of the doses, though they be small, is oppressed and overcome, and thus being disabled from calling into exercise the force of curative reaction, is compelled involuntarily to yield to the continuation of the excessive medicinal disease imposed upon it, in a manner similar to what is daily observed in the allœopathic abuse of large and accumulating doses of one and the same medicine, to the lasting injury of the patient.

Avoiding the errors here indicated, in order to arrive at the desired object with more certainty than heretofore, and so to administer the selected remedy that its virtues may be obtained without injury to the patient, that in a given case of disease all the benefit may be derived from it which, from its nature, it is capable of effecting, I have, of late, pursued a peculiar method.

I perceived that in order to discover the true medium path, it is necessary to be guided by the nature of the different medicines, as well as the bodily constitution of the patient, and the magnitude of his disease. Let us give an example in the use of *sulphur* in chronic (psoric) diseases. The most subtile dose of this remedy (*tinct. sulph.* X°), even in robust persons with developed psora, can seldom be advantageously repeated oftener than every seven days, and the interval is to be proportionably prolonged, when a more feeble and irritable patient of this kind is to be treated, to nine, twelve, or fourteen days, before the repetition of a similar dose ; but it is then to be repeated again and again as long as the same remedy continues to be serviceable. It is found (to continue the example of sulphur) that, in psoric diseases, seldom less than four, often six or eight, or even ten such doses (*tinct. sulph.* X°) are requisite for the complete destruction of that portion of the chronic disease which sulphur is capable of removing, to be administered in the aforesaid intervals—provided there has been no previous allœopathic abuse of that medicine. *Thus a (primary) psoric eruption of recent origin in a person not too much weakened, even when it may have extended over the whole body, can be thoroughly cured by means of a dose of sulphur repeated every seven days* within the space of ten to twelve weeks, (with ten to twelve of such globules,) so that it is rarely necessary, as an additional remedy, to administer a few doses of *carb. veg.* X° (in like manner given every week) *without any external treatment whatever, except a frequent change of linen, and appropriate regimen.*

When in other important chronic diseases, eight, nine, or ten doses of *tinct. sulph.* (X°) may be considered necessary, instead of administering them all in immediate succession, it is preferable, after each dose, or after every *two* or *three* doses, to interpose another suitable remedy which, after sulphur, is particularly homœopathic in the case, (mostly *hepar. sulph. calc.,*) and to permit this to operate for eight, nine, twelve, or fourteen days before a repetition of three doses of sulphur.

It not unfrequently happens, however, that the vital power rises in opposition to the action of many doses of sulphur, and will not permit the tranquil operation of this remedy even in the intervals above indicated, how necessary soever it may be for the chronic malady. This opposition is announced by some symptoms of the remedy, which, though moderate, yet become evident during the treatment. It is then sometimes advisable to administer a small dose of *nux vom.* X°, and suffer it to operate eight or ten days, in order to incline nature to permit the sulphur again to act in repeated doses, quietly and effectually. In fitting cases, *puls.* X° is to be preferred.

But the vital power offers the most resistance to the operation of sulphur, however plainly it may be indicated, when the remedy had been previously abused (even years before) in large doses. Here an aggravation of the chronic disease is conspicuous upon exhibiting the smallest dose of the remedy, even after smelling a globule moistened with *tinct. sulph.* X. This deplorable condition, which renders almost impossible the best medical treatment of chronic diseases, is one among the many which would lead us to bemoan the very general deterioration of chronic diseases, caused by the mal-practice of the old school, were we not here in possession of a remedy.

In such cases, let the patient once strongly smell a globule as large as a mustard seed, moistened with *hydrarg. met.* X, which is to be allowed to operate about nine days, in order to render the vital power again disposed for the beneficial operation of sulphur upon it (at least by the smelling of *tinct. sulph.* X°)—a discovery for which we are indebted to Dr. Griesselich, of Carlsruhe.

Of the other antipsoric remedies, (except, perhaps, *phosph.* X,) it will be necessary to administer a smaller number of doses at similar intervals, (of *sepia.* and *sil.* at longer intervals, without an intermediate remedy, where they are homœopathically indicated,) in order to destroy all that is curable by the remedy, in a given case. *Hep. sulph.* can rarely be given in substance or by smelling at shorter intervals than every fourteen or fifteen days.

It is presumed that previously to undertaking such a repetition of doses, the physician is well convinced that he has chosen the proper homœopathic remedy.

In acute diseases, the periods for repeating the dose must be regulated by the more or less rapid course of the disease to be combated, so that, when requisite, it may be given in twenty-four, sixteen, twelve, eight, or four hours, or even at shorter intervals, if without check, or the production of new symptoms, the remedy has proved beneficial; but for a dangerous acute disease whose progress is rapid, the interval must be lessened; thus in the most rapidly mortal disease with which we are acquainted, in cholera, one or two drops of a dilute solution of camphor must be administered every five minutes, in order to procure speedy and certain relief; and in the more developed form of the disease, doses of *cuprum veratrum, phosphor.*, &c. (X°), often every two to three hours, as well as *arsen. carb. veg.*, &c., at intervals equally short.

In the treatment of the so-called nervous fever, and other continued fevers, the practitioner is to be governed, in the repetition of the minutest dose of the suitable medicine, by the same precautions.

In pure syphilitic diseases I have generally found a single dose of mercury (X°) sufficient; yet where the least complication with psora was perceptible, sometimes two or three such doses were necessary, given in intervals of six or eight days.

In those cases wherein a particular remedy is strongly indicated, but the patient is very weak and irritable, once smelling a globule of the size of a mustard seed, moistened with the medicine, is safer and more serviceable than when it is taken in substance, even in the minutest dose of the higher dilutions. In the process of smelling, the patient should hold the vial containing the globule under one nostril, when one momentary inhalation of the air in the vial is to be made ; and if the dose is intended to be stronger, the same operation may be repeated with the other nostril. The operation of the medicine thus administered, continues as long as when it is taken in substance, and therefore the smelling must not be repeated at shorter intervals than when taken in the latter mode.

§ 247. Subject to these conditions, the most subtile doses of the best chosen homœopathic medicine can be repeated at intervals of fourteen, twelve, ten, eight, to seven days, with the best and frequently almost incredible effects ; when more haste is necessary, in cases of chronic disease approaching to acute, it may be repeated at still shorter intervals ; but in acute diseases, the periods of repetition may be far more considerably abridged to twenty-four, twelve, eight, or four hours ; and in the most acute, from one hour down to five minutes. In short, proportionably to the greater or less rapidity with which the disease runs its course, and to the nature of the remedy administered, as is more fully explained in the note to the preceding paragraph.

§ 248. The dose of the same medicine should be repeated until a cure is effected, or until it ceases any longer to afford relief; in the latter alternative, the remnant of the disease, with its altered group of symptoms, will require another homœopathic remedy.

§ 249. Every medicine which, in the course of its operation, produces new symptoms that do not appertain to the disease to be cured, and that are annoying, is incapable of procuring real amendment,* and cannot be considered as homœopathically chosen. If the deterioration of symptoms be important, the effect of the medicine must be extinguished, in part, without delay, by means of an antidote, before another and more homœopathic remedy is given; or, if the new symptoms be not violent, the other remedy must be immediately given, to take the place of that which has been so unfitly chosen.

* All experience teaches us, that scarcely any homœopathic medicine can be prepared in too minute a dose to produce perceptible benefit in a dis-

ease to which it is adapted. (§ 161. 279.) Hence it would be an improper and injurious practice, when the medicine produces no good effect, or an inconsiderable exacerbation of the symptoms, after the manner of the old school, to repeat or increase the dose under the idea that it cannot prove serviceable on account of its minuteness. Every exacerbation caused by new symptoms, when nothing injurious has occurred with regard to diet or mental impressions, always proves the unsuitableness of the medicine previously given, but never indicates the weakness of the dose.

§ 250. When in urgent cases, after the lapse of six, eight, to twelve hours, it becomes manifest to the observant physician who has accurately investigated the character of the disease, that he has made a false selection of the remedy last administered, when, during the appearance of new symptoms, the disease becomes, though slightly, yet evidently worse from hour to hour, it is not only admissible, but duty renders it imperative on him to rectify the mistake he has made, and administer another homœopathic remedy, not only tolerably, but the best possibly adapted to the morbid condition at the time (§ 167).

§ 251. There are some medicines, for example, ignatia amara, bryonia, rhus, and sometimes belladonna, whose power of changing the human economy chiefly consists in the production of alternate effects—a kind of primary symptoms, partly in opposition to each other. If the physician find no improvement after the strict homœopathic selection and administration of one of these remedies, (in acute cases, after a few hours,) then by repeating it in the same dilution, he will quickly obtain the desired effect.*

* As I have explained more circumstantially in the introduction to the article ignatia (Mat. Med. vol. ii.)

The signs of incipient amendment.

§ 252. But if in a chronic disease (psoric) the most homœopathic remedy, (antipsoric,) administered in the smallest and most suitable dose, does not produce an amendment, it is a sure sign that the cause which keeps up the disease still exists, and that there is something either in the regimen or condition of the patient that must be first altered before a permanent cure can be effected.

§ 253. In all diseases, particularly those which are acute,

the state of mind and general demeanour of the patient are among the first and most certain of the symptoms (which are not perceived by every one) that announce the beginning of any slight amendment or augmentation of the malady. If the disease begins to improve, though in ever so slight a degree, the patient feels more at ease, he is more tranquil, his mind is less restrained, his spirits revive, and all his conduct is, so to express it, more natural. The very reverse takes place where there is only a slight increase; an embarrassment and helplessness, which call for commiseration, are observable in the mind and temper of the patient, as well as in all his actions, gestures, and postures—something both remarkable and peculiar which cannot escape the eye of an attentive observer, but which it would be difficult to describe in words.*

* But the signs of amendment furnished by the mind and temper of the patient, are never visible, (shortly after he has taken the remedy,) but where the dose has been *attenuated to the proper degree*—that is to say, as much as possible. A dose stronger than necessary (even of the most homœopathic remedy) acts with too great violence, and plunges the moral and intellectual faculties into such disorder that it is impossible to discover quickly any amendment that takes place. I must observe in this place, that it is the common fault of physicians who go from the old school of medicine over to the homœopathic, to violate this most important rule. Blinded by prejudice, they avoid small doses of medicines attenuated to the highest degree, and thus deprive themselves of the great advantages which experience has a thousand times proved to result from them; they cannot accomplish that which the true homœopathist is capable of doing, and yet they falsely declare themselves his disciples.

§ 254. If we add to this, either the appearance of fresh symptoms, or the aggravation of those which previously existed, or, on the contrary, the diminution of the primitive symptoms without the manifestation of any new ones, the physician who is gifted with discrimination and discernment will no longer doubt whether the disease is aggravated or ameliorated, though there may be patients who are incapable of telling whether they are better or worse, and even some who refuse to tell it.

§ 255. Even in the latter case it is easy to arrive at the positive truth, by going through all the symptoms which have been noted down in the description of the malady and passing them in review successively with the patient. If the latter

does not complain of any new symptoms that were not mentioned before—if none of the previous symptoms are aggravated in a manifest degree—and when, finally, an amendment
of the moral and intellectual faculties is perceptible—it is certain that the remedy has effected an essential diminution of
the malady, or if only too short an interval has elapsed since
its administration, that it is on the point of doing so.   But if
the remedy has been well selected, and the amendment, notwithstanding, delays its appearance, it can only be attributed,
either to some irregularity on the part of the patient, or to the
lengthened duration of the homœopathic aggravation (§ 151)
excited by the medicinal substance, and we ought thence to
conclude that the dose was not minute enough.

§ 256.   On the other hand, if the patient describes any
recent symptoms of some importance, (which indicate the unsuitable choice of the remedy,) it will be vain for him to
declare that he feels himself better ; the physician, far from
believing him, ought, on the contrary, to consider him worse
than before, of the truth of which he will soon have ocular
demonstration.

Blind predilection for favourite remedies, and unjust aversion to others.

§ 257.   A true physician will beware of forming a predilection for any particular remedies which chance may sometimes have led him to administer with success.   This preference might cause him to reject others which would be still
more homœopathic, and consequently of greater efficacy.

§ 258.   He must, likewise, be careful not to entertain a
prejudice against those remedies from which he may have experienced some check, because he had made a bad selection ;
and he should never lose sight of this great truth, that of all
known remedies, there is but one that merits a preference
before all others, viz.—that whose symptoms bear the closest
resemblance to the totality of those which characterize the
malady.   No petty feeling should have any influence in so
serious a matter.

The regimen proper in chronic diseases.

§ 259.   As it is requisite, in the homœopathic treatment,
that the doses should be extremely small, it may be readily

conceived that everything which exercises a medicinal influence on the patient, should be removed from his *regimen and mode of life*, in order that the effects of such minute doses may not be destroyed, overpowered or disturbed, by any foreign stimulant.*

* The softest tones of the flute, which at a distance in the stillness of the night inspire the gentle mind with a sentiment of religion and piety, only cleave the air in vain when they are accompanied by noise and discordant sounds.

§ 260. In chronic diseases, more especially, it is important to remove all obstacles of this nature with the greatest care, since it is by them, or some other errors in regimen, (which often remain undiscovered,) that they are aggravated.*

* Such, for example, as by coffee, teas of all the different kinds, or beer containing vegetable substances that are unfit for the patient, liqueurs, (cordials,) especially those prepared from medicinal aromatics, all kinds of punch, spiced chocolate, sweet waters and perfumery of all kinds, odorous flowers in the room, preparations for the teeth either in powder or liquid wherein medicinal substances are included, perfumed bags, strongly seasoned viands and sauces, pastry and ice cream with aromatics, pot herbs, culinary greens, or roots containing medicinal properties, old cheese or butter, stale meat, the flesh and fat of swine, geese and ducks, young veal, or acids. Every one of these act medicinally, and ought to be carefully removed from patients of this kind. All excesses at table are to be interdicted, even in the use of sugar and salt, as well as of spirituous liquors, hot rooms, flannel worn next to the skin. (Flannel must not be left off till warm weather, and then exchanged for cotton, and afterwards for linen.) The physician will likewise forbid a sedentary life in close rooms, passive exercise, (by riding or driving, swinging and rocking in chairs,) sleeping too long after dinner, nocturnal occupations, uncleanliness, unnatural voluptuousness, and the reading of obscene books, the occasions of anger, grief, and malice, a passion for gaming, excessive mental and bodily labour, a residence in a marshy situation, or in a chamber that is not properly ventilated, penurious living, &c., &c. All practicable care should be observed by the patient to avoid these forbidden things, in order that no impediment may be interposed which would render the cure difficult or impossible. Some of my adherents appear to exact too much from their patients, by unnecessarily and improperly excluding from their diet things indifferent.

§ 261. The most suitable regimen in chronic diseases consists in removing everything which might impede the cure, and by bringing about an opposite state, where it is necessary, by recommending innocent cheerfulness, exercise in the open

air, in almost all weathers, (daily walks, light manual labour,)
aliments that are suitable, nourishing, and free from medicinal influence, &c., &c.

Regimen in acute diseases.

§ 262. On the other hand, in acute diseases, (mental alienation excepted,) the preservative instinct of the vital power
speaks in so clear and precise a manner that the physician has
only to recommend to the family or nurses of the patient not
to thwart nature by refusing the patient anything he may long
for, or by trying to persuade him to take things that might do
him injury.

§ 263. The food and drink demanded by a patient labouring under an acute disease, act for the most part as palliatives
only, and can at farthest effect momentary relief; but they
contain no real medicinal qualities, and are merely conformable to a species of desire on his part. Provided the gratification which they, in this respect, procure the patient, be
confined within proper limits, the slight obstacles* which they
could place in the way of a radical cure of the disease are
more than covered by the influence of the homœopathic remedy, by the greater extent of liberty given to the vital powers,
and the ease and satisfaction that follow the possession of any
object that is ardently desired. In acute diseases, the temperature of the chamber as well as the quantity of bed-covering
should likewise be regulated according to the wishes of the
patient; likewise care is to be taken to remove everything
that could disturb his mental repose.

* These are, however, unfrequent. Thus, for example, in a pure inflammatory disease, where aconite is indispensable, but which by the use of vegetable acids would be neutralized, the patient has, in almost all cases, a longing
for pure cold water.

On the choice of the purest and most energetic medicines.

§ 264. A skilful physician will never rely on the curative
virtues of medicines unless he has procured them in the *most
pure and perfect state.* It is, therefore, requisite that he should
be *capable of judging* of their purity.

§ 265. For the repose of his own conscience, he ought to

be thoroughly convinced that the patient always takes the right remedy chosen for him.

§ 266.   Substances derived from the animal and vegetable kingdoms are never in the full possession of their medicinal virtues but when they are in a raw state.*

* All animal and vegetable substances in a crude state are more or less possessed of medicinal virtues, and can modify the health each in its own peculiar manner.   The animals and plants which civilized nations are in the habit of using as food, have the advantage over all others, that they contain more nourishment, are less energetic in their medicinal properties, the greater part of which is lost by the preparation which they undergo—such as by the expression of the pernicious juice, (e. g. of the American cassada,) by fermentation, (that of the dough with which bread is made, sourcrout, &c. by dressing or torrefaction, which either destroys or dissipates the parts to which these properties adhere.   The addition of salt or vinegar likewise produces the same effect, but then other inconveniences result from it.
Plants containing the most powerful medicinal virtues are likewise rendered totally or partially inert when they are treated by the same process. Iris root, horseradish, the arum and peony, also become inert by drying. The virtues of the most active vegetable juices are often completely destroyed by the high temperature employed in the preparation of their extracts.   The juice of the most dangerous plant will be divested of all its properties if it be suffered to stand still for a certain time—it passes rapidly into a state of vinous fermentation even when the temperature is moderate, and immediately after it becomes sour, and then putrid, which annihilates all its medicinal virtues, and the sediment which remains is nothing more than inert fecula. Green herbs put together in a heap lose the greater part of their medicinal properties by the transudation which they undergo.

The mode of preparing the most energetic and durable medicines from fresh herbs.

§ 267.   The most certain and effectual means of obtaining the medicinal power of indigenous plants which can be procured fresh, is to express their juice and mix it immediately after with equal parts of alcohol of sufficient strength to consume spunk that is immersed in it.   Let the mixture stand twenty-four hours in corked bottles, decant the clear liquor from the filamentous and glairy dregs, then preserve for medicinal use.[1]   The alcohol which is added to the juice prevents fermentation.   The liquor is to be kept in a dark place in well-corked glass bottles.   In this manner the medicinal virtues of plants may be preserved for ever perfect and .ree from the slightest change.[2]

[1] Buchholz (Taschenbuch für Scheidekünstler und Apotheker, 1815, L.

VI.) assures his readers, (uncontradicted by his critic in the "Leipziger Litera-
turzeitung, 1816, No. 82,") that they are indebted to the Russian Campaign
for this excellent mode of preparing medicines, previous to which (1812) it
was unknown in Germany. But, in reporting this *in the very words* of the
first edition of my Organon, he intentionally conceals that I am the author
who published it two years before the Russian Campaign (1810.) Some
people would rather make it appear that a discovery came from the deserts
of Asia, than attribute the honour of it to a German! It is true, alcohol was
formerly sometimes added to the juice of plants in order to preserve it for a
time previous to making extracts of it ; but this addition was never made
with the intent of administering this mixture under the title of a remedy.

  ³ Although equal parts of alcohol and juice recently expressed are generally the proportions best suited to produce the precipitation of albuminous and
fibrous matter, there are, however, some plants which contain so much mucus, such as symphytum, jacea, &c., or an extraordinary quantity of albumen,
such as, athuca synapium, solanum nigrum, and others, that they usually require double the quantity of alcohol. As regards plants that are very dry,
such as, oleander, buxus, taxus, ledum, sabina, &c., it is necessary to commence by rubbing them down into a homogeneous and humid paste, and then
add double the quantity of alcohol, which unites with the vegetable juice, and
facilitates its extraction by means of the press. But the latter may be also
rubbed to the third power with sugar of milk, and afterwards its energy developed according to § 271.

Dry vegetable substances.

  § 268. With regard to exotic plants, bark, seeds, and roots,
which cannot be obtained in a fresh state, a prudent physician
will never accept the powder upon the faith of other individuals. Before he makes use of them in his practice, it is necessary that he should have them entire and unprepared, to be
able to satisfy himself of their purity.*

  * To preserve them in the form of powder, one precaution is necessary,
which has hitherto been neglected by the majority of pharmacopolists, who
were unable to preserve even the most carefully-dried animal and vegetable
substances in the form of powder without their undergoing a change. Vegetable substances, even when they are perfectly dry, still retain a certain portion of moisture which is indispensable to the cohesion of their tissue, which
does not prevent the drug being incorruptible so long as it is left entire, but
which becomes superfluous the moment it is pulverized. It therefore follows,
that any animal or vegetable substance that was quite dry when entire, becomes slightly moist when reduced to the form of powder, which soon spoils and
grows mouldy even in bottles that are well stopped, unless this superfluous
moisture has been previously removed. The best mode of effecting this is to
spread the powder on a flat plate of tin with raised edges, floating in a boiling
water-bath, and stir it till the parts no longer hang in small lumps, but glide

separately from each other like fine sand. When they are dried by this process, and sealed up in bottles, powders will retain all their primitive medicinal powers *for ever*, without either *growing mouldy or engendering mites*, but care must be taken to keep the bottles in a dark place enclosed in chests or boxes. Animal and vegetable substances gradually lose their medicinal virtues even when they are preserved entire, but much more so when they are in the form of powder, if the bottles are not stoppered air-proof, and kept in a dark place.

The homœopathic method of preparing crude medicinal substances, in order to obtain their greatest medicinal power.

§ 269. The homœopathic healing art develops for its purposes the immaterial (dynamic) virtues of medicinal substances, and, to a degree previously unheard of, by means of a peculiar and hitherto untried process. By this process it is that they become penetrating, operative, and remedial, even those that, in a natural or crude state, betrayed not the least medicinal power upon the human system.

§ 270. If two drops of a mixture of equal parts of alcohol and the recent juice of any medicinal plant (see § 267) be diluted with ninety-eight drops of alcohol in a vial capable of containing one hundred and thirty drops, and the whole twice shaken together, the medicine becomes exalted in energy (*potenzirt*) to the first development of power, or, as it may be denominated, the first potence. The process is to be continued through twenty-nine additional vials, each of equal capacity with the first, and each containing ninety-nine drops of spirits of wine; so that every successive vial, after the first, being furnished with one drop from the vial or dilution immediately preceding, (which had just been twice shaken,) is, in its turn, to be shaken twice,* remembering to number the dilution of each vial upon the cork as the operation proceeds. These manipulations are to be conducted thus through all the vials, from the first up to the thirtieth or decillionth development of power, (*potenzirte Decillion-Verdünnung, X.*), which is the one in most general use.

* In order to have a determinate rule for the moderate development of power of the fluid medicines, multiplied experience and observation have led me to retain two shakes for every vial, in preference to a greater number, which had previously been used, but which developed the energy in too great a degree. On the contrary, there are homœopathists who, in their visits to

15

the sick, carry about their persons the medicines in a fluid state, which, they nevertheless affirm, do not in time become increased in energy by the frequent agitation to which they are thus subjected. This declaration, however, betrays on their part the want of a talent for accurate observation. I dissolved a grain of natron in half an ounce of a mixture of water and a little alcohol, poured the solution into a vial, which was thereby filled two-thirds, and shook it uninterruptedly for half an hour. By this agitation, the fluid attained an energy equal to that of the thirtieth dilution.

§ 271. All other medicinal substances, excepting sulphur, which of latter years has been employed only in the form of . the highly diluted tincture (X), such, for example, as the metals, either pure, oxydized, or in the form of sulphurets, and other minerals, petroleum, phosphorus, the parts or juices of plants, obtainable only in their dry or inspissated state, animal substances, neutral salts, &c.—one and all were, in the first place, exalted in energy by attenuation in the form of powder, (by means of three hours' trituration in a mortar,) to the millionth degree. Of this, one grain was then dissolved and brought through twenty-seven vials, by a process similar to that employed in the case of vegetable juices, up to the thirtieth development of power.*

* The process is described at large in the " *Chronische Krankheiten*," second edition, and in the " *Arzneimittellehre*," vol. ii. third edition.

Only one simple *medicine to be administered at a time.*

§ 272. In no instance is it requisite to employ more than *one simple* medicinal substance at a time.*

* Experiments have been made by some homœopathists in cases where, imagining that one part of the symptoms of a disease required one remedy, and that another remedy was more suitable to the other part, they have given both remedies at the same time, or nearly so ; but I earnestly caution all my adherents against such a hazardous practice, which never will be necessary, though, in some instances, it may appear serviceable.

§ 273. It is scarcely possible to conceive how a doubt can still exist on the question, whether it is more reasonable and conformable to nature to employ but one known medicine at a time in a case of sickness, or to prescribe a mixture of several drugs.

§ 274. As the true physician finds in simple and uncompounded medicines all he can desire—that is to say, the artificial morbific agents whose homœopathic powers completely cure natural diseases; and as it is a wise precept never to attempt with the aid of several powers that which can be effected by a single one, he will never think of administering as a remedy more than one simple medicine at a time. For he knows that if even the pure and specific effects of every medicine upon the healthy state of man, had been discovered, we should still remain as ignorant as we were before, as to the manner in which two medicinal substances, mixed together, might oppose and modify each other reciprocally in their effects. He is aware that a single medicine, administered in a disease where the totality of the symptoms is perfectly similar to its own, cures it completely; and he is likewise convinced, even in the least favourable case, where the remedy would not perfectly harmonize with the malady, in regard to the resemblance of the symptoms, that it leads to a knowledge of the curative medicine, since the new symptoms which it excites in such a case confirm those which it formerly created, when tried upon healthy individuals—an advantage that can never be derived where compound medicines are employed.*

* A judicious physician will confine himself to an internal application of the remedy which he has selected as homœopathic as possible, and will leave the use of ptisans, little bags filled with medicinal herbs, fomentations of vegetable decoctions, washes, and frictions with different species of ointments, injections, &c., to those who practise according to routine.

Strength of the doses used in homœopathic treatment. The manner of graduating them, or of augmenting or diminishing their power. The development of their powers.

§ 275. The appropriation of a medicine to any given case of disease does not depend solely upon the circumstance of its being perfectly homœopathic, but also upon the minute quantity of the dose in which it is administered. If *too strong a* dose of a remedy, that is even entirely homœopathic, be given, it will infallibly injure the patient, though the medicinal substance be of ever so salutary a nature; the impression it makes is felt more sensibly, because, in virtue of its homœopathic character, the remedy acts precisely on those parts of the organism which have already been most exposed to the attacks of the natural disease.

§ 276. Even a homœopathic medicine is, on this account, always injurious when given in too large a dose, and hurtful to the patient in proportion to the extent of the quantity administered. But the increase of the dose itself is also prejudicial in the same degree as the remedy is more homœopathic; and a strong dose of such a medicine would do more harm than the dose of an allœopathic medicinal substance (which bears no analogy whatever to the disease) of equal strength; for, in that case, the homœopathic aggravation (§ 157—160)—that is to say, the artificial malady, which is very analogous to the natural one excited by the remedy in the most suffering parts of the organism—is carried to a height that is injurious (§ 246, note); whereas, if it had been confined within proper limits, it would have effected a gentle, prompt, and certain cure. It is true the patient no longer suffers from the primitive malady which has been homœopathically destroyed, but he suffers so much more from the medicinal one which was much too powerful, and from unnecessary debility.

§ 277. For this very reason, and because a remedy administered in a dose sufficiently small is so much more efficacious, nay, almost wonderfully so, in proportion as it has been homœopathically selected, in the same manner, a medicine whose peculiar symptoms correspond perfectly with those of the disease, ought to be salutary in proportion as the dose approaches nearer to the appropriate minuteness to which it should be reduced to effect a gentle cure.

§ 278. The question that now suggests itself is, to discover what may be the degree of minuteness of the dose best calculated to render the salutary effects intended to be produced certain, and gentle—that is to say, how far the dose of a homœopathic remedy, in any given case of disease, ought to be reduced, in order to derive from it the best possible cure. It may be readily conceived that no theoretical conjecture will furnish an answer to this problem, and that it is not by such means we can establish, in respect to each individual medicine, the quantity of the dose that suffices to produce the homœopathic effect, and accomplish a prompt and gentle cure. No reasonings, however ingenious, will avail in this instance. It is by pure experiments only, and precise observations, that this object can be attained. It would be absurd to bring forward as an objection the large doses used in ordinary medicine, which are not applied to the suffering parts themselves, but merely to those not attacked by the disease. This would be no argument against the minuteness of the doses which pure experiments have proved to be necessary in homœopathic treatment.

§ 279. It has been *fully* proved by pure experiments, that when a disease does not evidently depend upon the impaired state of an important organ, even though it were of a chronic nature, and complicated, and due care has been taken to remove from the patient all foreign medicinal influence, *the dose of the homœopathic remedy can never be sufficiently small so as to be inferior to the power of the natural disease which it can, at least, partially extinguish and cure, provided it be capable of producing only a small increase of symptoms immediately after it is administered.* (§ 157—160.)

§ 280. This incontrovertible axiom, founded upon experience, will serve *as a rule by which the doses of all homœopathic medicines, without exception, are to be attenuated to such a degree, that after being introduced into the body they shall merely produce an almost insensible aggravation of the disease.* It is of little import whether the attenuation goes so far as to appear almost impossible to ordinary physicians whose minds feed on no other ideas but what are gross and material.* All their arguments and vain assertions will be of little avail when opposed to the dictates of unerring experience.

* Mathematicians will inform them, that in whatever number of parts they may divide a substance, each portion still retains a *small share* of the material; that, consequently, the most diminutive part that can be conceived never ceases to be *something*, and can, in no instance, be reduced to nothing. Physicians may learn from them that there exist immense powers which have no weight, such as light and heat, and which are consequently infinitely lighter than the medicinal contents of the smallest homœopathic doses. Let them weigh, if they can, the injurious words which excite a bilious fever, or the afflicting news of the death of a son, which terminates the existence of an affectionate mother. Let them only touch, for a quarter of an hour, a magnet capable of carrying a weight of an hundred pounds, and the pain will soon teach them that even the imponderable bodies can also produce on man the most violent medicinal effects! Let any of these weak-minded mortals of a de-

licate constitution but gently apply, during a few minutes, to the pit of the
stomach the extremity of the thumb of a vigorous mesmerist who has fixed
his intent, and the disagreeable sensations that he experiences will soon
make him repent having set limits to the boundless activity of nature.

If the allœopathist, in essaying the homœopathic method, cannot resolve
upon administering doses that are so feeble and attenuated, only let him ask
himself what risk he ventures by doing so. If there is nothing real except
that which is possessed of weight, and if everything which has no weight
ought to be looked upon as equal to nothing, a dose that appears to him like
nothing, could have no worse results than that of producing no effect at all,
which is at least far more innocent than the effects resulting from the strong
doses of allœopathic medicines. Why will the physician believe his own in-
experience, which is flanked by prejudice, more competent than the experience of several years grounded upon facts ? Added to this, the homœopathic
medicines acquire at each division or dilution a new degree of power by the
rubbing or shaking they undergo, a means of developing the inherent virtues
of medicines that was unknown till my time ; and which is so energetic, that
latterly I have been forced by experience to reduce the number of shakes to
two, of which I formerly prescribed *ten* to each dilution.

§ 281. All diseases have an extraordinary tendency to undergo a change when operated upon by the influence of
homogeneous medicinal agents. There is no patient, however
robust his constitution may be, who, if attacked merely by a
chronic disease, or by what is called a local malady, does not
speedily experience a favourable change in the suffering parts
after having taken the appropriate homœopathic remedy in
the smallest dose possible. In short, the effects of this substance will make a greater impression on him than they
would upon a healthy child twenty-four hours after its birth.
How insignificant and ridiculous is mere theoretic incredulity,
when opposed to the infallible evidence of facts !

§ 282. However feeble the dose of a remedy may be, provided it can in the slightest degree aggravate the state of the
patient homœopathically,—provided it has the power of exciting symptoms similar to those of the primitive disease, but
rather more intense,—it will, in preference, and almost exclusively, affect those parts of the organism that are already in a
state of suffering, and which are strongly irritated and predis-
posed to receive any irritation analogous to their own. Thus
an artificial disease rather more intense is substituted in the
place of the natural one. The organism no longer suffers but
from the former affection, which, by reason of its nature, and

the minuteness of the dose by which it was produced, soon yields to the efforts of the vital force to restore the normal state, and thus leaves the body (if the disease was an acute one) free from suffering—that is to say, in a healthy condition.

§ 283. To proceed, therefore, in a manner conformable to nature, the true physician will only administer a homœopathic remedy in the precise dose necessary to exceed and destroy the disease to which it is opposed, so that if by one of those errors, pardonable to human frailty, he had made choice of a remedy that was inappropriate, the injury that might result from it would be so slight that the development of the vital force, and the administration of the smallest dose of another remedy more homœopathic, would suffice to repair it.

§ 284. The effects of a dose are by no means diminished in the same proportion as the quantity of the medicinal substance is attenuated in the homœopathic practice. Eight drops of a tincture taken at once do not produce upon the human body *four times* the effect of a dose of two drops ; they merely produce one that is nearly double. In the same manner the *single drop* of a mixture, composed of one drop of a tincture and ten of a liquid void of all medicinal properties, does not produce *ten times* the effect that a drop ten times more attenuated would produce, but merely an effect that is scarcely *double*. The progression continues according to this law, so that a single drop of a dilution, attenuated in the highest degree, ought, and does in fact, produce a very considerable effect.*

* Suppose, for example, that one drop of a mixture containing the tenth of a grain of any medicinal substance produces an effect $= a$; a drop of another mixture containing merely a hundredth part of a grain of this same substance will only produce an effect $= \frac{a}{2}$; if it contains a ten thousandth part of a grain of medicine, the effect will be $= \frac{a}{4}$; if a millionth, it will be $= \frac{a}{8}$; and so on progressively, to an equal volume of the doses ; the effects of the remedy on the body will merely be diminished about one half each time that the quantity is reduced nine-tenths of what it was before. I have often seen a drop of the tincture of nux vomica at the *decillionth* degree of dilution, produce exactly half the effect of another at the *quintillionth* degree, when I administered both one and the other to the same individual, and under the same circumstances.

§ 285. By diminishing the volume of the dose, the power of it is also diminished; that is to say, when instead of one entire drop of attenuated tincture, merely a fraction of this drop be administered,* the object of rendering the effect less powerful is then very perfectly attained. The reason of this may be easily conceived : the volume of the dose being diminished, it must necessarily follow that it will touch a less number of the nerves of the living organism, by contact with which, it is true, the power of the medicine is communicated to the whole body, but it is transmitted in a smaller degree.

---

* The best mode of administration is to make use of small globules of sugar, the size of a mustard seed ; one of these globules having imbibed the medicine, and being introduced into the vehicle, forms a dose containing about the three hundredth part of a drop, for three hundred of such globules will imbibe one drop of alcohol ; by placing one of those on the tongue, and not drinking anything after it, the dose is considerably diminished. But if the patient is very sensitive, and it is necessary to employ the smallest dose possible, and attain at the same time the most speedy results, it will be sufficient to let him smell once. (See § 288, note.)

§ 286. For the same reason, the effect of a homœopathic dose is increased when we augment the quantity of the liquid in which it is dissolved to administer it to the patient ; but then the remedy comes in contact with a much more extended surface, and the nerves that feel its effects are far more numerous. Although theorists have asserted that the extension of a medicine in liquid weakens its action, experience proves the reverse, at least as far as regards homœopathic remedies.*

---

* Only wine and alcohol, which are the most simple of all excitants, lose a portion of their heating and exciting power when they are attenuated in a large quantity of water.

§ 287. It ought, however, to be observed, that there is a wide difference between mixing imperfectly the medicinal substance with a certain quantity of liquid, and incorporating it so intimately[1] that the smallest fraction of the liquid may still retain a proportion of the medicine equal to that which exists in all the others. In short, the mixture possesses a much greater medicinal power in the second case than it does

in the first. Rules may be deduced from this to serve as a
guide in the preparation of homœopathic medicines, where it
is necessary to diminish the effects of the remedies as much as
possible in order to make them supportable to the most delicate patients.[2]

[1] When I make use of the word *intimately*, I mean to say that by shaking
a drop of medicinal liquid with ninety-nine drops of alcohol once—that is to
say, by taking the phial in the hand which contains the whole, and imparting
to it a rapid motion by a single powerful stroke of the arm descending, I shall
then obtain an exact mixture of them; but that two, three, or ten such movements would render the mixture much closer—that is to say, they would develop the medicinal virtues still further, making them, as it were, more
potent, and their action on the nerves more penetrating. In proceeding,
therefore, to the dilution of medicinal substances, it is wrong to give the
twenty or thirty successive attenuating glasses more than two shakes, where
it is merely intended to develop the power of the medicines in a moderate
degree. It would also be well in the attenuation of powders not to rub them
down too much in the mortar; thus, for example, when it is requisite to mix
one grain of a medicinal substance in its entire state with ninety-nine grains of
sugar of milk, it ought to be rubbed down with force during one hour only,
and the same space of time should not be exceeded in the subsequent tritura-
tions, in order that the power of the medicine may not be carried to too great
an extent. More ample instructions on this head are to be found in the first
part of my work on chronic diseases, second edition.

[2] The higher the dilutions of a medicine are carried in the process of developing its power by means of twice shaking, the more rapidly and with the
more penetrating influence does it appear to affect medicinally the vital power,
and produce changes in the economy with an energy but little diminished, even
if the process of dilution be carried to a great extent; for instance, instead of
the ordinary dilution X, (which is mostly sufficient,) it be carried up to XX,
L, C, and even higher dilutions.

What parts of the body are more or less sensible to the action of medicines.

§ 288. The action of medicines in a liquid form* upon the
body is so penetrating, it propagates itself with so much rapidity and in a manner so general, from the irritable and sensitive part which has undergone the first impression of the medicinal substance to all the other parts of the body, that we
might almost call it a spiritual (dynamic or virtual) effect.

* Homœopathic remedies operate with the most certainty and energy by
smelling or inhaling the medicinal aura constantly emanating from a saccha-

rine globule that has been impregnated with the higher dilution of a medicine, and in a dry state enclosed in a small vial. One globule (of which 10, 20 to 100 weigh a grain) moistened with the 30th dilution and then dried, provided it be preserved from heat and the light of the sun, retains its virtues undiminished, at least for eighteen or twenty years, (so far my experience extends,) although the vial that contained it had during that time been opened a thousand times. Should the nostrils be closed by coryza or polypus, the patient may inhale through his mouth, holding the mouth of the vial between his lips. It may be applied to the nostrils of small children while they are asleep with the certainty of success. During these inhalations the medicinal aura comes in contact with the nerves, which are spread over the parietes of the ample cavities through which it freely passes, and thus influences the vital power in the mildest yet most powerful and beneficial manner. All that is curable by homœopathy may with the most certainty and safety be cured by this mode of receiving the medicine. Of late I have become convinced of the fact, (which I would not have previously believed,) that smelling imparts a medicinal influence as energetic and as long-continued as when the medicine is taken in substance by the mouth, and at the same time that its operation is thus more gentle than when administered by the latter mode. It is therefore requisite that the intervals for repeating the smelling should not be shorter than those prescribed for taking the medicine in a more substantial form.

§ 289. Every part of the body that is sensible to the touch is equally susceptible of receiving the impression of medicines and of conveying it to all the other parts.

§ 290. Next to the stomach, the tongue and mouth are the parts most susceptible of receiving medicinal influence. However, the interior of the nose, the intestinum rectum, the genitals, and all parts endowed with great sensibility, are equally susceptible of the influence of medicines. This is the reason that when the latter are introduced into the body through wounds or ulcers, they act as energetically as if administered by the mouth.

§ 291. Even those organs which have lost the sense that was peculiar to them—such, for example, as the tongue and palate deprived of taste, the nose of smell, &c.—communicate to all the other parts of the body the effects of the medicines acting immediately on themselves, in as perfect a manner as if they were in possession of their own peculiar faculties.

§ 292. Although the surface of the body is covered with skin and epidermis, it is not less accessible to the action of medicines, especially of such as are liquid. However, the most sensitive parts of this covering are those which have the greatest tendency to receive it.*

* Rubbing appears only to favour the action of the medicine so far as it renders the skin more sensitive, and the living fibre more apt, not only to feel in a certain extent the medicinal virtue, but also to communicate the sensation to the whole of the economy. After having rubbed the inner part of the thighs once, it will suffice afterwards merely to lay the mercurial ointment on the parts, to obtain the same medicinal result as if direct friction had been used. What is called "rubbing in" is of questionable utility, as it is not certain whether the metal in substance can, by this process, penetrate the interior of the body, or be taken up by the lymphatic vessels. The homœopathist has little to do with *rubbing*, and makes no use whatever of mercurial ointments in his method of cure.

Animal magnetism (mesmerism). On the application of positive and negative mesmerism.

§ 293. I again find it necessary, in this place, to say a few words on the subject of animal magnetism, the nature of which differs so greatly from that of all other remedies. This curative power, (which should be called *mesmerism*, after the name of its inventor, *Mesmer*,) of whose efficacy none but madmen can entertain a doubt, which, through the powerful will of a well-intentioned individual, influences the body of the patient by the touch, acts homœopathically by exciting symptoms analogous to those of the malady—and this object is attained by a single transit, the determination being moderately fixed, and gliding the hands slowly over the body from the crown of the head to the soles of the feet.[1] In this form it is applicable to internal hemorrhages in their last stage, when they threaten death. It acts likewise by imparting a uniform degree of vital power to the organism when there is an excess of it at one point and a deficiency at another—such, for example, as where there is a determination of blood to the head, or when a patient, in a state of debility, is subject to insomnolency, anxiety, &c. In this case, a single transit, similar to the preceding one, but stronger, is to be practised.

Finally, it acts by immediately communicating a degree of vital power to a weak part or to the entire organism—an effect that cannot be produced by any other means with such certainty, and without interfering with the other medical treatment. This third indication is performed by assuming a very firm and decided manner, and applying the hands or tips of the fingers to the weak part, which an internal chronic affection has made the seat of its principal local symptom— such, for example, as old ulcers, amaurosis, paralysis of a limb, &c.[2] To this class belong certain apparent cures that have, in all ages, been performed by magnetisers who were endowed with great natural strength. But the most brilliant result of the communication of human vigour to the entire organism is where, by the resolute and fixed determination of a man in the full vigour of life,[3] it recalls to life persons who have remained in a state of apparent death during a long interval of time,—a species of resurrection of which history records many examples.

[1] The smallest homœopathic dose, when properly applied, effects wonders. It not unfrequently occurs, that patients are overwhelmed, by incompetent homœopathists, with a rapid succession of remedies, which, though well selected and of the highest potence, yet produce a state of such excessive irritability, that the life of the patient is placed in jeopardy, and another dose, however mild, may prove fatal. Uuder such circumstances, the hand of the mesmeriser, gently sliding down, and frequently touching the part affected, produces an uniform distribution of the vital power through the system, and rest, sleep, and health, are restored.

[2] Although this operation of locally supplying the vital power, which ought to be occasionally repeated, cannot effect a durable cure when the local affection is of an ancient date, and depends upon (what very frequently occurs) some general internal malady, still the positive communication of the vital power, which is no more a palliative than food and drink to hunger and thirst, is of no slight aid in the radical cure of the entire affection by antipsoric remedies.

[3] Particularly one of those men, of whom there are but few, who, possessing great goodnature and complete bodily power, have a *very moderate inclination for sexual intercourse*, and are able without difficulty to suppress all their desires ; in whom, consequently, an abundance of the subtle vital energy, which would else be employed in the secretion of semen, is disposed to communicate itself to other men through the medium of the touch, seconded by a strong intention of the mind. Some such powerful mesmerisers whom I have known had all these singular peculiarities.

§ 294. All these methods of applying mesmerism depend upon the afflux of a greater or lesser quantity of vital power in the body of the patient, and are, on that account, termed positive mesmerism.[1] But there exists yet another, which deserves the name of negative mesmerism, because it produces a contrary effect. To this class belong the customary transits to awaken a subject from a state of somnambulism, and all the manual operations which are designated by the names *calming* and *ventilating*. The most simple and certain means of discharging, by the aid of negative mesmerism, the excess of vital power accumulated in any part of the body of a patient who has not been weakened, consist in passing, in a rapid manner, the right arm, extended at about the distance of an inch from the body, from the crown of the head to the soles of the feet.[2] The quicker this passage is performed, the stronger is the discharge that it produces. It can, for example, when a woman, previously in the enjoyment of health,[3] has been plunged into a state of apparent death by the suppression of her menses occasioned by some violent mental commotion, recall her to life by carrying off the vital power which probably accumulated in the precordial region, and reestablish the equilibrium in the whole organism.[4] In the same manner a slight negative passage, that is less rapid, frequently allays the great agitation and fatiguing insomnolency which are the results of a positive passage that is too strong when exercised upon a very irritable patient.

[1] In treating here of the certain and decided curative virtues of positive mesmerism, I do not speak of the frequent abuses that are made of it, where, by repeating the passages during half an hour, and even a whole hour, daily, they occasion, in patients labouring under nervous affections, that vast revolution of the human economy which bears the name of *somnambulism*—a state in which man, removed from the animal world, appears to belong more to the spiritual world, a highly unnatural and dangerous condition, by means of which a cure of chronic diseases has frequently been attempted.

[2] It is a known rule, that a person subjected to either positive or negative mesmerism, ought not to wear silk on any part of the body.

[3] Consequently, a negative transit, particularly if it is very rapid, would be extremely injurious to a person who had been for any length of time in a weak condition, or in whom the vital powers were not very active.

[4] A young country boy of robust constitution, about ten years of age, was mesmerised for some slight indisposition by a woman who performed several

strong passages on him with the ends of her two thumbs, from the precordial region down to the termination of the ribs; the boy immediately fell pale as death into such a state of insensibility and immobility, that all means were tried in vain to recall him to life, and he was thought to be dead. I caused his elder brother to make as rapid a transit as possible on him from the crown of the head to the soles of the feet; he immediately recovered his senses, and was healthy and cheerful.

THE END.

CPSIA information can be obtained at www.ICGtesting.com
Printed in the USA
LVOW10*0851041014

407284LV00005B/43/P